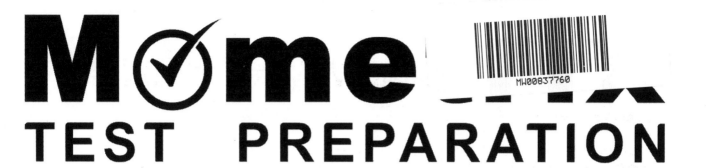

Mome

TEST PREPARATION

Secrets of the

ARDMS

Ultrasound Physics & Instrumentation Exam Study Guide

DEAR FUTURE EXAM SUCCESS STORY

First of all, **THANK YOU** for purchasing Mometrix study materials!

Second, congratulations! You are one of the few determined test-takers who are committed to doing whatever it takes to excel on your exam. **You have come to the right place.** We developed these study materials with one goal in mind: to deliver you the information you need in a format that's concise and easy to use.

In addition to optimizing your guide for the content of the test, we've outlined our recommended steps for breaking down the preparation process into small, attainable goals so you can make sure you stay on track.

We've also analyzed the entire test-taking process, identifying the most common pitfalls and showing how you can overcome them and be ready for any curveball the test throws you.

Standardized testing is one of the biggest obstacles on your road to success, which only increases the importance of doing well in the high-pressure, high-stakes environment of test day. Your results on this test could have a significant impact on your future, and this guide provides the information and practical advice to help you achieve your full potential on test day.

Your success is our success

We would love to hear from you! If you would like to share the story of your exam success or if you have any questions or comments in regard to our products, please contact us at **800-673-8175** or **support@mometrix.com**.

Thanks again for your business and we wish you continued success!

Sincerely,
The Mometrix Test Preparation Team

Need more help? Check out our flashcards at:
http://MometrixFlashcards.com/ARDMS

TABLE OF CONTENTS

Introduction

Thank you for purchasing this resource! You have made the choice to prepare yourself for a test that could have a huge impact on your future, and this guide is designed to help you be fully ready for test day. Obviously, it's important to have a solid understanding of the test material, but you also need to be prepared for the unique environment and stressors of the test, so that you can perform to the best of your abilities.

For this purpose, the first section that appears in this guide is the **Secret Keys**. We've devoted countless hours to meticulously researching what works and what doesn't, and we've boiled down our findings to the five most impactful steps you can take to improve your performance on the test. We start at the beginning with study planning and move through the preparation process, all the way to the testing strategies that will help you get the most out of what you know when you're finally sitting in front of the test.

We recommend that you start preparing for your test as far in advance as possible. However, if you've bought this guide as a last-minute study resource and only have a few days before your test, we recommend that you skip over the first two Secret Keys since they address a long-term study plan.

If you struggle with **test anxiety**, we strongly encourage you to check out our recommendations for how you can overcome it. Test anxiety is a formidable foe, but it can be beaten, and we want to make sure you have the tools you need to defeat it.

Secret Key 1: Plan Big, Study Small

There's a lot riding on your performance. If you want to ace this test, you're going to need to keep your skills sharp and the material fresh in your mind. You need a plan that lets you review everything you need to know while still fitting in your schedule. We'll break this strategy down into three categories.

Information Organization

Start with the information you already have: the official test outline. From this, you can make a complete list of all the concepts you need to cover before the test. Organize these concepts into groups that can be studied together, and create a list of any related vocabulary you need to learn so you can brush up on any difficult terms. You'll want to keep this vocabulary list handy once you actually start studying since you may need to add to it along the way.

Time Management

Once you have your set of study concepts, decide how to spread them out over the time you have left before the test. Break your study plan into small, clear goals so you have a manageable task for each day and know exactly what you're doing. Then just focus on one small step at a time. When you manage your time this way, you don't need to spend hours at a time studying. Studying a small block of content for a short period each day helps you retain information better and avoid stressing over how much you have left to do. You can relax knowing that you have a plan to cover everything in time. In order for this strategy to be effective though, you have to start studying early and stick to your schedule. Avoid the exhaustion and futility that comes from last-minute cramming!

Study Environment

The environment you study in has a big impact on your learning. Studying in a coffee shop, while probably more enjoyable, is not likely to be as fruitful as studying in a quiet room. It's important to keep distractions to a minimum. You're only planning to study for a short block of time, so make the most of it. Don't pause to check your phone or get up to find a snack. It's also important to **avoid multitasking**. Research has consistently shown that multitasking will make your studying dramatically less effective. Your study area should also be comfortable and well-lit so you don't have the distraction of straining your eyes or sitting on an uncomfortable chair.

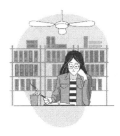

The time of day you study is also important. You want to be rested and alert. Don't wait until just before bedtime. Study when you'll be most likely to comprehend and remember. Even better, if you know what time of day your test will be, set that time aside for study. That way your brain will be used to working on that subject at that specific time and you'll have a better chance of recalling information.

Finally, it can be helpful to team up with others who are studying for the same test. Your actual studying should be done in as isolated an environment as possible, but the work of organizing the information and setting up the study plan can be divided up. In between study sessions, you can discuss with your teammates the concepts that you're all studying and quiz each other on the details. Just be sure that your teammates are as serious about the test as you are. If you find that your study time is being replaced with social time, you might need to find a new team.

Secret Key 2: Make Your Studying Count

You're devoting a lot of time and effort to preparing for this test, so you want to be absolutely certain it will pay off. This means doing more than just reading the content and hoping you can remember it on test day. It's important to make every minute of study count. There are two main areas you can focus on to make your studying count.

Retention

It doesn't matter how much time you study if you can't remember the material. You need to make sure you are retaining the concepts. To check your retention of the information you're learning, try recalling it at later times with minimal prompting. Try carrying around flashcards and glance at one or two from time to time or ask a friend who's also studying for the test to quiz you.

To enhance your retention, look for ways to put the information into practice so that you can apply it rather than simply recalling it. If you're using the information in practical ways, it will be much easier to remember. Similarly, it helps to solidify a concept in your mind if you're not only reading it to yourself but also explaining it to someone else. Ask a friend to let you teach them about a concept you're a little shaky on (or speak aloud to an imaginary audience if necessary). As you try to summarize, define, give examples, and answer your friend's questions, you'll understand the concepts better and they will stay with you longer. Finally, step back for a big picture view and ask yourself how each piece of information fits with the whole subject. When you link the different concepts together and see them working together as a whole, it's easier to remember the individual components.

Finally, practice showing your work on any multi-step problems, even if you're just studying. Writing out each step you take to solve a problem will help solidify the process in your mind, and you'll be more likely to remember it during the test.

Modality

Modality simply refers to the means or method by which you study. Choosing a study modality that fits your own individual learning style is crucial. No two people learn best in exactly the same way, so it's important to know your strengths and use them to your advantage.

4

For example, if you learn best by visualization, focus on visualizing a concept in your mind and draw an image or a diagram. Try color-coding your notes, illustrating them, or creating symbols that will trigger your mind to recall a learned concept. If you learn best by hearing or discussing information, find a study partner who learns the same way or read aloud to yourself. Think about how to put the information in your own words. Imagine that you are giving a lecture on the topic and record yourself so you can listen to it later.

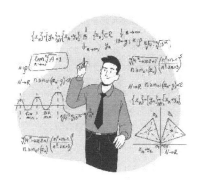

For any learning style, flashcards can be helpful. Organize the information so you can take advantage of spare moments to review. Underline key words or phrases. Use different colors for different categories. Mnemonic devices (such as creating a short list in which every item starts with the same letter) can also help with retention. Find what works best for you and use it to store the information in your mind most effectively and easily.

Secret Key 3: Practice the Right Way

Your success on test day depends not only on how many hours you put into preparing, but also on whether you prepared the right way. It's good to check along the way to see if your studying is paying off. One of the most effective ways to do this is by taking practice tests to evaluate your progress. Practice tests are useful because they show exactly where you need to improve. Every time you take a practice test, pay special attention to these three groups of questions:

- The questions you got wrong
- The questions you had to guess on, even if you guessed right
- The questions you found difficult or slow to work through

This will show you exactly what your weak areas are, and where you need to devote more study time. Ask yourself why each of these questions gave you trouble. Was it because you didn't understand the material? Was it because you didn't remember the vocabulary? Do you need more repetitions on this type of question to build speed and confidence? Dig into those questions and figure out how you can strengthen your weak areas as you go back to review the material.

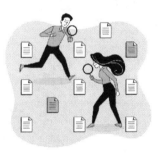 Additionally, many practice tests have a section explaining the answer choices. It can be tempting to read the explanation and think that you now have a good understanding of the concept. However, an explanation likely only covers part of the question's broader context. Even if the explanation makes perfect sense, **go back and investigate** every concept related to the question until you're positive you have a thorough understanding.

As you go along, keep in mind that the practice test is just that: practice. Memorizing these questions and answers will not be very helpful on the actual test because it is unlikely to have any of the same exact questions. If you only know the right answers to the sample questions, you won't be prepared for the real thing. **Study the concepts** until you understand them fully, and then you'll be able to answer any question that shows up on the test.

It's important to wait on the practice tests until you're ready. If you take a test on your first day of study, you may be overwhelmed by the amount of material covered and how much you need to learn. Work up to it gradually.

On test day, you'll need to be prepared for answering questions, managing your time, and using the test-taking strategies you've learned. It's a lot to balance, like a mental marathon that will have a big impact on your future. Like training for a marathon, you'll need to start slowly and work your way up. When test day arrives, you'll be ready.

Start with the strategies you've read in the first two Secret Keys—plan your course and study in the way that works best for you. If you have time, consider using multiple study resources to get different approaches to the same concepts. It can be helpful to see difficult concepts from more than one angle. Then find a good source for practice tests. Many times, the test website will suggest potential study resources or provide sample tests.

Practice Test Strategy

If you're able to find at least three practice tests, we recommend this strategy:

UNTIMED AND OPEN-BOOK PRACTICE

Take the first test with no time constraints and with your notes and study guide handy. Take your time and focus on applying the strategies you've learned.

TIMED AND OPEN-BOOK PRACTICE

Take the second practice test open-book as well, but set a timer and practice pacing yourself to finish in time.

TIMED AND CLOSED-BOOK PRACTICE

Take any other practice tests as if it were test day. Set a timer and put away your study materials. Sit at a table or desk in a quiet room, imagine yourself at the testing center, and answer questions as quickly and accurately as possible.

Keep repeating timed and closed-book tests on a regular basis until you run out of practice tests or it's time for the actual test. Your mind will be ready for the schedule and stress of test day, and you'll be able to focus on recalling the material you've learned.

Secret Key 4: Pace Yourself

Once you're fully prepared for the material on the test, your biggest challenge on test day will be managing your time. Just knowing that the clock is ticking can make you panic even if you have plenty of time left. Work on pacing yourself so you can build confidence against the time constraints of the exam. Pacing is a difficult skill to master, especially in a high-pressure environment, so **practice is vital**.

Set time expectations for your pace based on how much time is available. For example, if a section has 60 questions and the time limit is 30 minutes, you know you have to average 30 seconds or less per question in order to answer them all. Although 30 seconds is the hard limit, set 25 seconds per question as your goal, so you reserve extra time to spend on harder questions. When you budget extra time for the harder questions, you no longer have any reason to stress when those questions take longer to answer.

Don't let this time expectation distract you from working through the test at a calm, steady pace, but keep it in mind so you don't spend too much time on any one question. Recognize that taking extra time on one question you don't understand may keep you from answering two that you do understand later in the test. If your time limit for a question is up and you're still not sure of the answer, mark it and move on, and come back to it later if the time and the test 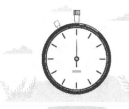 format allow. If the testing format doesn't allow you to return to earlier questions, just make an educated guess; then put it out of your mind and move on.

On the easier questions, be careful not to rush. It may seem wise to hurry through them so you have more time for the challenging ones, but it's not worth missing one if you know the concept and just didn't take the time to read the question fully. Work efficiently but make sure you understand the question and have looked at all of the answer choices, since more than one may seem right at first.

Even if you're paying attention to the time, you may find yourself a little behind at some point. You should speed up to get back on track, but do so wisely. Don't panic; just take a few seconds less on each question until you're caught up. Don't guess without thinking, but do look through the answer choices and eliminate any you know are wrong. If you can get down to two choices, it is often worthwhile to guess from those. Once you've chosen an answer, move on and don't dwell on any that you skipped or had to hurry through. If a question was taking too long, chances are it was one of the harder ones, so you weren't as likely to get it right anyway.

On the other hand, if you find yourself getting ahead of schedule, it may be beneficial to slow down a little. The more quickly you work, the more likely you are to make a careless mistake that will affect your score. You've budgeted time for each question, so don't be afraid to spend that time. Practice an efficient but careful pace to get the most out of the time you have.

Secret Key 5: Have a Plan for Guessing

When you're taking the test, you may find yourself stuck on a question. Some of the answer choices seem better than others, but you don't see the one answer choice that is obviously correct. What do you do?

The scenario described above is very common, yet most test takers have not effectively prepared for it. Developing and practicing a plan for guessing may be one of the single most effective uses of your time as you get ready for the exam.

In developing your plan for guessing, there are three questions to address:

- When should you start the guessing process?
- How should you narrow down the choices?
- Which answer should you choose?

When to Start the Guessing Process

Unless your plan for guessing is to select C every time (which, despite its merits, is not what we recommend), you need to leave yourself enough time to apply your answer elimination strategies. Since you have a limited amount of time for each question, that means that if you're going to give yourself the best shot at guessing correctly, you have to decide quickly whether or not you will guess.

Of course, the best-case scenario is that you don't have to guess at all, so first, see if you can answer the question based on your knowledge of the subject and basic reasoning skills. Focus on the key words in the question and try to jog your memory of related topics. Give yourself a chance to bring the knowledge to mind, but once you realize that you don't have (or you can't access) the knowledge you need to answer the question, it's time to start the guessing process.

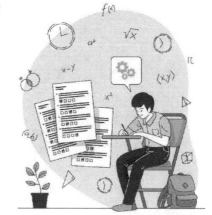

It's almost always better to start the guessing process too early than too late. It only takes a few seconds to remember something and answer the question from knowledge. Carefully eliminating wrong answer choices takes longer. Plus, going through the process of eliminating answer choices can actually help jog your memory.

Summary: Start the guessing process as soon as you decide that you can't answer the question based on your knowledge.

10

How to Narrow Down the Choices

The next chapter in this book (**Test-Taking Strategies**) includes a wide range of strategies for how to approach questions and how to look for answer choices to eliminate. You will definitely want to read those carefully, practice them, and figure out which ones work best for you. Here though, we're going to address a mindset rather than a particular strategy.

Your odds of guessing an answer correctly depend on how many options you are choosing from.

Number of options left	5	4	3	2	1
Odds of guessing correctly	20%	25%	33%	50%	100%

You can see from this chart just how valuable it is to be able to eliminate incorrect answers and make an educated guess, but there are two things that many test takers do that cause them to miss out on the benefits of guessing:

- Accidentally eliminating the correct answer
- Selecting an answer based on an impression

We'll look at the first one here, and the second one in the next section.

To avoid accidentally eliminating the correct answer, we recommend a thought exercise called **the $5 challenge**. In this challenge, you only eliminate an answer choice from contention if you are willing to bet $5 on it being wrong. Why $5? Five dollars is a small but not insignificant amount of money. It's an amount you could

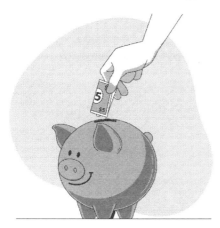

afford to lose but wouldn't want to throw away. And while losing $5 once might not hurt too much, doing it twenty times will set you back $100. In the same way, each small decision you make—eliminating a choice here, guessing on a question there—won't by itself impact your score very much, but when you put them all together, they can make a big difference. By holding each answer choice elimination decision to a higher standard, you can reduce the risk of accidentally eliminating the correct answer.

The $5 challenge can also be applied in a positive sense: If you are willing to bet $5 that an answer choice *is* correct, go ahead and mark it as correct.

Summary: Only eliminate an answer choice if you are willing to bet $5 that it is wrong.

Which Answer to Choose

You're taking the test. You've run into a hard question and decided you'll have to guess. You've eliminated all the answer choices you're willing to bet $5 on. Now you have to pick an answer. Why do we even need to talk about this? Why can't you just pick whichever one you feel like when the time comes?

The answer to these questions is that if you don't come into the test with a plan, you'll rely on your impression to select an answer choice, and if you do that, you risk falling into a trap. The test writers know that everyone who takes their test will be guessing on some of the questions, so they intentionally write wrong answer choices to seem plausible. You still have to pick an answer though, and if the wrong answer choices are designed to look right, how can you ever be sure that you're not falling for their trap? The best solution we've found to this dilemma is to take the decision out of your hands entirely. Here is the process we recommend:

Once you've eliminated any choices that you are confident (willing to bet $5) are wrong, select the first remaining choice as your answer.

Whether you choose to select the first remaining choice, the second, or the last, the important thing is that you use some preselected standard. Using this approach guarantees that you will not be enticed into selecting an answer choice that looks right, because you are not basing your decision on how the answer choices look.

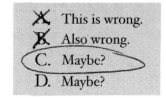

This is not meant to make you question your knowledge. Instead, it is to help you recognize the difference between your knowledge and your impressions. There's a huge difference between thinking an answer is right because of what you know, and thinking an answer is right because it looks or sounds like it should be right.

Summary: To ensure that your selection is appropriately random, make a predetermined selection from among all answer choices you have not eliminated.

Test-Taking Strategies

This section contains a list of test-taking strategies that you may find helpful as you work through the test. By taking what you know and applying logical thought, you can maximize your chances of answering any question correctly!

It is very important to realize that every question is different and every person is different: no single strategy will work on every question, and no single strategy will work for every person. That's why we've included all of them here, so you can try them out and determine which ones work best for different types of questions and which ones work best for you.

Question Strategies

⊘ READ CAREFULLY

Read the question and the answer choices carefully. Don't miss the question because you misread the terms. You have plenty of time to read each question thoroughly and make sure you understand what is being asked. Yet a happy medium must be attained, so don't waste too much time. You must read carefully and efficiently.

⊘ CONTEXTUAL CLUES

Look for contextual clues. If the question includes a word you are not familiar with, look at the immediate context for some indication of what the word might mean. Contextual clues can often give you all the information you need to decipher the meaning of an unfamiliar word. Even if you can't determine the meaning, you may be able to narrow down the possibilities enough to make a solid guess at the answer to the question.

⊘ PREFIXES

If you're having trouble with a word in the question or answer choices, try dissecting it. Take advantage of every clue that the word might include. Prefixes and suffixes can be a huge help. Usually, they allow you to determine a basic meaning. *Pre-* means before, *post-* means after, *pro-* is positive, *de-* is negative. From prefixes and suffixes, you can get an idea of the general meaning of the word and try to put it into context.

⊘ HEDGE WORDS

Watch out for critical hedge words, such as *likely, may, can, sometimes, often, almost, mostly, usually, generally, rarely*, and *sometimes*. Question writers insert these hedge phrases to cover every possibility. Often an answer choice will be wrong simply because it leaves no room for exception. Be on guard for answer choices that have definitive words such as *exactly* and *always*.

⊘ SWITCHBACK WORDS

Stay alert for *switchbacks*. These are the words and phrases frequently used to alert you to shifts in thought. The most common switchback words are *but, although*, and *however*. Others include *nevertheless, on the other hand, even though, while, in spite of, despite*, and *regardless of*. Switchback words are important to catch because they can change the direction of the question or an answer choice.

⊘ FACE VALUE

When in doubt, use common sense. Accept the situation in the problem at face value. Don't read too much into it. These problems will not require you to make wild assumptions. If you have to go beyond creativity and warp time or space in order to have an answer choice fit the question, then you should move on and consider the other answer choices. These are normal problems rooted in reality. The applicable relationship or explanation may not be readily apparent, but it is there for you to figure out. Use your common sense to interpret anything that isn't clear.

Answer Choice Strategies

⊘ ANSWER SELECTION

The most thorough way to pick an answer choice is to identify and eliminate wrong answers until only one is left, then confirm it is the correct answer. Sometimes an answer choice may immediately seem right, but be careful. The test writers will usually put more than one reasonable answer choice on each question, so take a second to read all of them and make sure that the other choices are not equally obvious. As long as you have time left, it is better to read every answer choice than to pick the first one that looks right without checking the others.

⊘ ANSWER CHOICE FAMILIES

An answer choice family consists of two (in rare cases, three) answer choices that are very similar in construction and cannot all be true at the same time. If you see two answer choices that are direct opposites or parallels, one of them is usually the correct answer. For instance, if one answer choice says that quantity x increases and another either says that quantity x decreases (opposite) or says that quantity y increases (parallel), then those answer choices would fall into the same family. An answer choice that doesn't match the construction of the answer choice family is more likely to be incorrect. Most questions will not have answer choice families, but when they do appear, you should be prepared to recognize them.

⊘ ELIMINATE ANSWERS

Eliminate answer choices as soon as you realize they are wrong, but make sure you consider all possibilities. If you are eliminating answer choices and realize that the last one you are left with is also wrong, don't panic. Start over and consider each choice again. There may be something you missed the first time that you will realize on the second pass.

⊘ Avoid Fact Traps

Don't be distracted by an answer choice that is factually true but doesn't answer the question. You are looking for the choice that answers the question. Stay focused on what the question is asking for so you don't accidentally pick an answer that is true but incorrect. Always go back to the question and make sure the answer choice you've selected actually answers the question and is not merely a true statement.

⊘ Extreme Statements

In general, you should avoid answers that put forth extreme actions as standard practice or proclaim controversial ideas as established fact. An answer choice that states the "process should be used in certain situations, if…" is much more likely to be correct than one that states the "process should be discontinued completely." The first is a calm rational statement and doesn't even make a definitive, uncompromising stance, using a hedge word *if* to provide wiggle room, whereas the second choice is far more extreme.

⊘ Benchmark

As you read through the answer choices and you come across one that seems to answer the question well, mentally select that answer choice. This is not your final answer, but it's the one that will help you evaluate the other answer choices. The one that you selected is your benchmark or standard for judging each of the other answer choices. Every other answer choice must be compared to your benchmark. That choice is correct until proven otherwise by another answer choice beating it. If you find a better answer, then that one becomes your new benchmark. Once you've decided that no other choice answers the question as well as your benchmark, you have your final answer.

⊘ Predict the Answer

Before you even start looking at the answer choices, it is often best to try to predict the answer. When you come up with the answer on your own, it is easier to avoid distractions and traps because you will know exactly what to look for. The right answer choice is unlikely to be word-for-word what you came up with, but it should be a close match. Even if you are confident that you have the right answer, you should still take the time to read each option before moving on.

General Strategies

⊘ Tough Questions

If you are stumped on a problem or it appears too hard or too difficult, don't waste time. Move on! Remember though, if you can quickly check for obviously incorrect answer choices, your chances of guessing correctly are greatly improved. Before you completely give up, at least try to knock out a couple of possible answers. Eliminate what you can and then guess at the remaining answer choices before moving on.

⊘ Check Your Work

Since you will probably not know every term listed and the answer to every question, it is important that you get credit for the ones that you do know. Don't miss any questions through careless mistakes. If at all possible, try to take a second to look back over your answer selection and make sure you've selected the correct answer choice and haven't made a costly careless mistake (such as marking an answer choice that you didn't mean to mark). This quick double check should more than pay for itself in caught mistakes for the time it costs.

⊘ Pace Yourself

It's easy to be overwhelmed when you're looking at a page full of questions; your mind is confused and full of random thoughts, and the clock is ticking down faster than you would like. Calm down and maintain the pace that you have set for yourself. Especially as you get down to the last few minutes of the test, don't let the small numbers on the clock make you panic. As long as you are on track by monitoring your pace, you are guaranteed to have time for each question.

⊘ Don't Rush

It is very easy to make errors when you are in a hurry. Maintaining a fast pace in answering questions is pointless if it makes you miss questions that you would have gotten right otherwise. Test writers like to include distracting information and wrong answers that seem right. Taking a little extra time to avoid careless mistakes can make all the difference in your test score. Find a pace that allows you to be confident in the answers that you select.

⊘ Keep Moving

Panicking will not help you pass the test, so do your best to stay calm and keep moving. Taking deep breaths and going through the answer elimination steps you practiced can help to break through a stress barrier and keep your pace.

Final Notes

The combination of a solid foundation of content knowledge and the confidence that comes from practicing your plan for applying that knowledge is the key to maximizing your performance on test day. As your foundation of content knowledge is built up and strengthened, you'll find that the strategies included in this chapter become more and more effective in helping you quickly sift through the distractions and traps of the test to isolate the correct answer.

Now that you're preparing to move forward into the test content chapters of this book, be sure to keep your goal in mind. As you read, think about how you will be able to apply this information on the test. If you've already seen sample questions for the test and you have an idea of the question format and style, try to come up with questions of your own that you can answer based on what you're reading. This will give you valuable practice applying your knowledge in the same ways you can expect to on test day.

Good luck and good studying!

Sound

For any medical imaging modality, a fundamental energy unit must be defined. Around this unit, the processes of energy production, interaction with the target, energy reception, and image formation will be carried out. In the case of ultrasound, the fundamental energy unit is the sound wave. Sound is a naturally occurring mechanism that we as humans perceive on a daily basis. It has been harnessed quite ingeniously by ultrasonic devices to produce an image of part of the human body. The understanding of sound and its behavior is the first step in understanding how ultrasound works.

Before sound can be defined, the concept of a medium must first be defined. A medium is simply any large volume of matter; examples of media are air, water, and in the case of ultrasound, body tissue. Each is made up of infinitely many subunits, or "particles," that are perceived to be evenly spaced and motionless relative to each other. The concept of a medium is fairly simple, as humans we are continuously surrounded by a medium of air that contains subunits of nitrogen, hydrogen, and oxygen. However, the presence of a medium is critical in ultrasound imaging because sound *requires* a medium, that is sound cannot exist in a vacuum. The properties of a given medium also heavily influence the manner in which sound moves or propagates through it.

A sound wave can be envisioned as an organized series of interruptions. The nature of these "interruptions" is an oscillation in the constituent particles of the medium, causing them to alternately be positioned closer to and farther apart from each other. The oscillations and therefore the sound wave must be produced by a source, will cross its medium in a straight line until a target is reached. A tuning fork is the easiest source to imagine, it physically oscillates back and forth causing adjacent air molecules to oscillate with it.

This movement causes a shift in several physical properties of the medium. The most significant of these is pressure, which undergoes local compression and rarefraction in a regular, alternating pattern. Graphically, pressure as a function of time for a given point in a medium through which sound propagates will appear as a sine wave.

However, recall that the sound wave is not stationary but propagates across its medium; while one area of the medium is compressed, the area ahead of it in the medium becomes rarefracted. For this point, rarefraction must be followed by compression, so the sound wave "moves" one step forward. If we were to set a fixed time and observe a larger section of the entire medium, a graph of pressure with respect to *distance* would also appear as a sine wave.

In combining these two ideas, we see that the true, full appearance of sound is that of a "moving" sine wave. The cause of this movement is the manner in which adjacent points in the medium oscillate at slight offsets to each other. Consider as an

19

example the ripples generated by throwing a rock into a pond. A snapshot of the surface of the water at a given time would reveal a sinusoidal pattern, while a close-up of a single location on the pond extended over a period of time would also reveal a sinusoidal pattern. The overall appearance is of moving waves propagating outwards from the point of contact.

WAVE EQUATION

Several variables are used to visualize and quantify the sound wave, many of which come from standard trigonometry. The two most important in terms of ultrasound are amplitude and frequency. For this application, amplitude is the change in pressure from rest to maximum compression or from rest to maximum rarefraction. Similarly, the "cycle" used in calculating frequency is the process of shifting from maximum compression to maximum rarefraction and back to maximum compression; the length of time for this cycle to occur is called the period. Frequency then is calculated as 1/period and is a measure of how "fast" the oscillations occur.

A standard format for expressing these two variables when describing a sound wave is known as the *wave equation.*

$$S(t) = A\cos(\omega t + \theta)$$

In this equation, sound is represented by S, as a function of time t; amplitude is represented by A, frequency is represented by ω (generally in radians/sec), and phase is represented by θ. Phase will be discussed in the forthcoming section. Note that sound could also be represented as a function of position rather than time.

The audible range for humans is from 20Hz to 20kHz; the greater the frequency of sound waves the higher its pitch will be. Other animals might have a wider audible range, this is why "dog whistles" don't bother us. The term "ultrasound" specifically refers to sound waves above 20kHz and thus above the audible range of humans. In ultrasound imaging the sound waves used to acquire images of the body range typically from 2 - 10Mhz, well outside of our audible range.

QUANTITATIVE PROPERTIES

In addition to the basic properties of amplitude and frequency, there are several other variables that help to define a sound wave. These variables can be divided into three categories, each of which describe a dimension spanned by sound:

- **Time**
  - Period - amount of time required for one cycle to pass. Also equal to the inverse of frequency, and measured in seconds.
  - Phase - amount of offset or delay. This can be expressed with respect to the origin or with respect to another waveform of equal frequency, and is measured as a fraction of the full period.

- **Space**
  - Speed - rate at which one point of the waveform (usually the front) progresses through the medium. This is a function of the properties of the medium and is expressed as a distance over time, usually m/s.
  - Wavelength - similar to the period, but in the spatial domain. The wavelength describes the distance covered by one cycle of the waveform as it progresses through the medium. It is calculated as the speed times the period. Again, period is the duration of one oscillation while wavelength is the length of one oscillation.
- **Magnitude**
  - Intensity - more commonly used instead of amplitude in order to quantify the magnitude of displacement imposed by a sound wave. Intensity is equal to the power carried by the sound wave averaged over a given period of time.

Power $=$ force $\times$ displacement/time

Power $=$ force exerted by pressure wave $\times$ medium velocity

$$\text{Intensity} = \frac{\text{Vmax}^2}{2Z}$$

- It represents how "loud" the sound is, and is expressed in decibels.

The above variables are summarized in the following table:

Variable	Symbol	Unit
Period	T	seconds
Phase	θ	radians
Speed	v	meters/second
Wavelength	λ	meters
Intensity	I	decibels

PULSE-MODE

The sound wave has until this point been described as a continuous sine wave, logically this form of ultrasound transmission is known as "continuous-mode". While this description represents sound in its truest and most natural form, an alternate method of sound generation is used more commonly in ultrasound and is known as "pulse-mode" or "pulsed ultrasound." Pulse-mode is preferred over continuous-mode because it takes better advantage of the properties of sound as applied to image formation, and because it simplifies the processes of sound generation and detection.

As the name would indicate, a "pulse" is a short burst of sound containing only a few cycles. A very basic pulse could be generated by turning your stereo on and then off very quickly. In pulse-mode ultrasound, the transducer is triggered such that it generates pulses of sound at set time intervals. The mechanisms of generation and means of quantification of the sound wave are fundamentally the same, except that the "down time" in between pulses must be factored in. Each pulse itself is made up of several sound waves, each of different frequency, superimposed upon each other and lasting for only a few cycles; the multiple-frequency composition allows the pulse to carry more information than would a single-frequency pulse when it comes time to reconstruct the received image.

In analyzing the entire signal that is output from the transducer, each pulse is viewed as a single, discrete unit. Rather than treating one full cycle of the continuous sine wave as an "event" as in the case of continuous-mode ultrasound, we now treat one pulse as an "event." Thus, the same quantifiers used to describe the oscillations in continuous mode are translated to describe the pulses in pulsed-mode. For example:

1. <u>Pulse repetition frequency</u> - The number of pulses that occur in one second.
2. <u>Pulse repetition period</u> - The amount of time in between pulses, that is the duration of the pulse itself plus the duration of the ensuing quiet period.
3. <u>Pulse duration</u> - The length of time required for only the pulse itself to be transmitted.
4. <u>Duty factor</u> - The fraction of "noisy time" to "quiet time", or pulse duration divided by pulse repetition period.

The purpose of pulse-mode will become clearer as we examine the interaction of sound with its surrounding medium and the methods by which transmitted sound is used to construct an image. The benefits of having discrete, separable bursts of sound rather than a single continuous signal will then become more apparent.

Mechanisms of Sound Generation

The physical generation of sound requires the displacement of particles that comprise the surrounding medium back and forth in order to generate the previously described waveform in an adjustable manner. Such an activity requires a device known as a transducer. In the case of ultrasound wave generation, the initial form of energy used by the transducer is a controlled electrical voltage, and the final form of energy is mechanical movement. This is a unique form of transduction; materials that can perform it are termed piezoelectric. Piezoelectricity can occur naturally in certain substances; most commonly, quartz crystals exist having an electrical construction that causes reshaping when an external voltage is applied. This reshaping pushes the air molecules surrounding the crystals in such a manner that sound is produced. Other piezoelectric elements have been artificially produced via the polarization of a ferroelectric material followed by heating and then slow cooling in the presence of an electric field; these are known as polarized ferroelectrics. Both natural and artificial piezoelectric elements use electric dipoles in their construction that realign under the presence of an applied voltage, causing the element to reshape.

The piezoelectric crystals used in ultrasound are flat and circular in shape and vibrate at a natural resonant frequency when electrically stimulated. That is, applying a voltage of varying magnitude will cause a sound of varying intensity to be produced, however this sound will be of a set frequency. Resonant frequency is inversely proportional to crystal thickness, therefore in order to change the frequency of the sound generated, a piezoelectric crystal of different thickness must be used. Transducers may be manipulated in ultrasound in many different ways in order to control their effects, for example while a single piezoelectric crystal makes up a *single-element transducer*; several crystals can be joined together to form a *multiple-element transducer*. The benefits of using multiple elements will be later explored.

While the piezoelectric crystal makes up the heart of the transducer, several other elements must also be included to ensure proper function. As we will see, the air-tissue interface in front of the face of the transducer will cause much of the transmitted energy from the piezoelectric element to be reflected back at the transducer, therefore a matching layer is used to mimic the properties of tissue and reduce or eliminate this interface. Backing material is used to reduce unwanted vibration, echoes, or backwardly-transmitted sound that would cause noise in the transducer. Especially in the case of pulse-mode ultrasound, the transducer must be able to generate short, distinct sound waves. The backing material essentially allows it to turn on and off quickly, without any lingering vibration. These elements are all contained within the transducer housing. External connections allow electrical stimulation of the electrodes, which of course cause movement of the piezoelectric crystal, ultimately resulting in the generation of sound.

BEAM FORMATION

While a sound wave comprises a single straight line of activity that moves through its medium, in Ultrasound practice many sound waves are used together, encompassing a certain thickness called a "beam." Similar to the light of a flashlight, a sound beam can be visualized as the region in front of the transducer that can receive or "hear" the sound wave, within which objects can be imaged. Immediately in front of the transducer, this region would have the shape of the transducer face; at farther depths the profile changes significantly. The shape of the beam is highly dependent on properties of its transducer; specifically, the two properties that affect beam profile are radius and resonant frequency. Resonant frequency is a function of the transducer's thickness; thus, the "output" can be completely controlled by the physical dimensions of the piezoelectric crystal.

The behavior of the ultrasound beam obeys Huygens' Principle, that is the beam generated by the entire source (transducer) may be considered as the sum of the beams generated by an infinite number of point sources. In the case of sound, each point source generates sound equally in all directions creating a spherical wave. The summation of these spherical waves forms the beam profile.

As you can see, the beam initially converges, in a region called the near field, and then diverges through the region known as the far field, up to infinity. These two regions are quantified as follows

$$\text{Near Field Length (NFL)} = \frac{a^2}{\Lambda}$$

$$\text{Far Field Divergence Angle} = (\theta)$$

$$\theta = \sin^{-1}\frac{(.61 \times \lambda)}{a}$$

where a is the radius of the transducer. Recall that λ, or wavelength, is a function of the speed of sound in the medium - a constant - and transducer frequency. Adjustment either of the two major quantifiers - radius or frequency - will allow for full control over the beam profile. While a single-element transducer of course cannot change its diameter, a multiple-element transducer can effectively do so by turning on or off the elements around its perimeter. An increase in diameter will cause an increase in the length of the near field and a decrease in the angle of divergence throughout the far field; these dimensions factor into the lateral resolution and focusing of the device.

The convergence angle of the near field is controlled by a lens placed in front of the transducer, which serves to focus the beam. Without a lens, sound would propagate outwards equally in all directions, rendering the transducer useless in terms of ultrasound. However, with a concave acoustic lens, the individual sound beams are deflected inwards throughout the Near Field Length. The cause of the beam's divergence at the end of the near field is unknown, however the result is that the beam thickness is at a minimum at medium distances, an area called the focal region. This region is the optimum length for obtaining an image from the sound wave, thus techniques are used by ultrasound designers to allow adjustment of the focal region onto the area of interest.

In addition to a piezoelectric crystal and an acoustic lens, the transducer contains two other elements that aid in maximizing its efficiency at generating a pure sound beam to be used in imaging the body. The first is a backing element, which is placed on the side of the transducer across from the beam to be generated. The purpose of the backing element is to absorb vibration from the transducer and remove any sound directed backwards, as these serve no useful purpose. The second item is a matching layer, which is placed in front of the piezoelectric crystal on the side of the beam. Its purpose is to serve as an intermediary between the surface of the piezoelectric element and the surface to be imaged; as we will see the drastically different properties of these two surfaces could cause problems without this intermediary.

PHASE STEERING

As the mechanics of the transducer can be manipulated to alter the dimensions of the sound beam, they can also be manipulated to alter the *direction* of the sound beam or beams. By using a multiple-element transducer, the time delay or phase offset of the various sound waves can be adapted such that the beam profiles generated by the transducer match a given application. For example, taking into account Huygens' Principle, consider a linear array in which each piezoelectric element sitting next in line is electrically stimulated after an appropriate delay. The net effect, as you can see, is a steered beam that leaves the transducer at an angle. Or, the same linear array can be fired such that the outer elements are stimulated before the inner elements, leading to a focused beam. The phase offset of multiple element transducers is one more variable that can be manipulated in the refinement of the ultrasound beam towards a specific application.

Sound Propagation/Interaction with Target

EFFECTS OF MEDIUM/TISSUE

At the start of image acquisition sound is produced by a transducer, introduced into a medium, and allowed to propagate. The events that occur during this period of propagation are functions of the target medium and its components but are fairly predictable. If the medium is a bucket of water, the sound wave will propagate in a straightforward manner at a constant speed and direction; its properties will change very little with distance as the medium is uniform. However, in ultrasound applications the medium in question is the human body, which is very non-uniform and contains multiple elements. As a result, the projected sound wave will interact with the target medium in various haphazard yet calculable ways, ultimately a return signal or signals will end up back at the transducer. The principle interactions that take place between the sound wave and its medium are classified as attenuation and reflection, both of which can be demonstrated by the simple example of standing across a football field from a friend and having him or her shout at you. Two effects will be recognized: first, the farther away your friend is, the harder it will be to hear him -- attenuation. Second an echo can be heard very shortly after the initial shout -- reflection.

ATTENUATION

The first of these effects is known as attenuation, an event that occurs in every medium (in the above example, the medium is air). Simply put, the intensity of a sound wave decreases with distance. As sound propagates, the particle oscillations that it causes require energy, causing the wave to lose energy mostly in the form of heat. The wave's intensity is a unitless quantity that is often taken to be unity at the transducer; because intensity only decreases at any point afterward it can be compared fractionally to its initial value. When expressed in decibels (further explained below), the rate of attenuation becomes a linear function, that is each time the sound wave covers a certain distance, a set amount of decrease in intensity will occur. This relationship does not change within the medium, it is a property specific to each different type of medium and is quantified by a variable called the attenuation coefficient. The larger the attenuation coefficient, the more rapidly the intensity of the sound wave will decrease. Air has a relatively small attenuation coefficient, which is why you would still hear your friend at the other end of a football field (a relatively large distance). Water, conversely, has a high attenuation coefficient. If your same friend was shouting at you underwater in a large pool, you would have a harder time hearing. As a general rule of thumb, a value of 1 dB per cm per MHz is used to define the attenuation of an ultrasound in soft tissue.

REFLECTION

The second effect demonstrated in the example, the echo, is a result of a phenomenon known as reflection. Reflection too is an easily understood event that

26

requires two adjacent media in which sound propagates. Reflection occurs at the interface between the two media with the amount of reflection depending on the acoustic impedance of the two media. Impedance is a difficult property to comprehend, mathematically it is equal to the product of two other material properties: density, which is the weight per given volume, and acoustic velocity, which specifies the speed at which sound naturally propagates through the material.

$$\text{Impedance} = \text{density} \times \text{velocity}$$

Impedance is equal to a resistance to movement; however, this has an inverse effect on the sound wave. Materials with a higher acoustic impedance will allow sound to pass through faster. Since acoustic velocity is a set property and is nearly the same for all biological tissue (with bone being an exception), impedance is essentially directly proportional to density.

Now that impedance has been (loosely) defined, the process of reflection can be examined within the context of an ultrasound wave propagating through body tissue. Reflection of sound in a medium is exactly what the name would imply - upon striking an interface, a sound wave will "bounce" back and propagate in the opposite direction.

An interface therefore is defined as the surface joining two adjacent mediums having different impedance values. It acts much like a wall that causes thrown tennis balls to bounce off of it. In fact, most interfaces within the body are caused by the walls of tissue or organs whose impedances differ from their surroundings. However, upon reaching a typical interface the sound wave will not be reflected entirely, only a fraction of it will bounce back while the remainder will continue to pass in the original direction and into the second medium. The two partial sound waves will have decreased pressure amplitude relative to the initial sound wave.

DB NOTATION

Unlike frequency, which is a numerically calculable and measurable quantity, the magnitude of the sound wave is essentially a unitless term. While it is possible to measure the degree of displacement of particles created by a given sound wave, the general convention used instead is to define some level of magnitude as a standard unit and to relate any other given magnitude as a fraction of this standard unit. In practice, these fractional terms can span a range of exponential proportions, so the decibel format is used.

One decibel is an arbitrary magnitude that has been chosen as the standard, base unit for sound and incorporated into everyday use. For example, the volume of a person whispering is equal to 30dB, the volume of a normal conversation stands at around 60dB, while the volume of a jet plane launching represents 130dB. In the case of ultrasound, however, volume (i.e. magnitude) is generated at an initial level and then *decreases* from there on. The same relationship will apply, only that each new magnitude X expressed in dB will now be a negative term due to the fact that the fraction X/S is less than one.

In addition to simplicity of terms, another advantage of using the decibel format in ultrasound is the compression of the integer range or expansion of the fractional range. The magnitude of sound covers an enormous dynamic range. Use of the decibel format shrinks this to a more manageable range; for example, the difference between 1dB and 100dB is a factor of 100,000. The opposite is true of the fractional range; an extremely small dynamic range is expanded by using the decibel convention.

REFRACTION

We have described how a sound wave will reflect off of a flat, perpendicular interface back towards its origin. Unfortunately, the majority of surfaces encountered in the body do not meet these criteria, that is, they are irregularly shaped and oddly positioned, which of course causes some complications. First consider a sound wave striking a non-perpendicular surface/interface, i.e. striking a flat interface at a given angle of incidence. Much like a pool ball striking a rail, this incident beam will be reflected away from the surface at an angle equal to its angle of incidence, away from the normal line. The departure angle, or angle of reflection, is equal to the angle of incidence. As in the case of a perpendicular incident beam, the reflected beam represents a fraction of the incident beam while the remainder, or transmitted beam, continues in its original direction. The transmitted beam simultaneously undergoes another process known as refraction. Refraction is caused by the differential impedance across the interface. As the sound beam, which spans a certain width, strikes this interface at a non-perpendicular angle it is slowed at a rate not uniform across its width, causing redirection. The same phenomenon can be observed by sticking a spear into a bucket of water: the spear appears to enter the water at a certain angle, then continue through underneath the water at a different angle. The spear does not actually bend, but the light waves that are perceived by the eye do, again caused by the change in impedance. While the reflected beam travels at an angle θ_r that is equal to the incident angle θ_i, the angle of the transmitted beam θ_t relates to the incident angle in a manner proportionate to the acoustic velocity of the two mediums. This behavior is governed by a set of equations similar to that of simple perpendicular reflection, with the angles accounted for. However, due to an interesting phenomenon, for an incident beam approaching above a critical angle θ_{ic}, complete reflection will occur.

SCATTER

Again, we must shift our attention from the ideal to the real in order to introduce a phenomenon present in ultrasound. No medium in the body is completely homogenous, and no surface is completely flat. Both of these properties lead to scatter, which occurs when small imperfections cause seemingly random reflections and refractions of the sound wave in all directions. This can exist in two forms: rough surfaces at impedance boundaries or suspended particles in the medium. Scatter is caused by *small* imperfections; small by definition is a term relative to the wavelength of the sound beam. Since a higher frequency waveform has a smaller wavelength, the imperfections in the surrounding medium will be larger relative to it, and it will be subject to a larger amount of scatter. In addition to frequency, the amount of scatter that will occur is dependent on the number of scatterers, the average size of the scatterers, and the amount of impedance difference between the scatterers and its surrounding or adjacent medium. While these imperfections do not greatly degrade the properties of the sound beam, their effects are significant enough to warrant mention.

Single Line Reconstruction

As has been described, a sound wave pulse projected into a medium will partially reflect back towards its generating transducer upon striking any interface within the medium. These interfaces generally occur at boundaries between different tissue types being imaged. The job of the transducer is not only to generate the initial sound pulse but to subsequently listen for reflected sound pulses striking its surface. Upon "hearing" the echoes, it must convert these pulses into electrical signals that are later reconstructed to form an image. Reflected pulses are the backbone of ultrasound: when an ultrasound image is displayed it is the *interfaces* that serve as data points to be visualized. To understand how a received sequence of echo pulses is used to reconstruct a complete image outlining the layout of tissue within the body, it is easiest to first consider a single one-dimensional strip of medium, which conceptually represents the area covered by a single sound wave.

The multiple interfaces in the path of the transducer and the sound pulse it generates will create a received signal consisting of a series of reflected pulses, or echoes. These echoes can be graphed with respect to time as shown below:

An echo is defined by two pieces of information: time and magnitude. Each is relative to the transmitted pulse at the transducer: time represents the duration of the period beginning at initial sound pulse generation, continuing through its reflection by a given interface, and finally concluding at its reception back at the transducer. Since there are multiple interfaces off of which the transmitted beam can reflect, multiple echoes will result from a single transmitted pulse. Magnitude represents the intensity of the received echo pulse as a fraction of the intensity of the initial sound pulse. Time and magnitude data are used together to back-calculate information about the interfaces that caused each echo. First, time can be translated into the distance from transducer to interface. Such a relationship depends simply on the acoustic velocity of the medium; assuming this to be constant, a time-distance proportionality is now defined. Second, the magnitude of the echo indicates the degree of impedance mismatch on either side of the interface. Larger impedance mismatches cause a larger fraction of the transmitted sound pulse to be reflected, and therefore cause a larger echo. Since the surrounding medium is usually assumed to be that of known impedance (i.e. water), when the amount of impedance mismatch is known the impedance of the tissue across the first interface encountered can be calculated. At each ensuing interface downstream, the same information is known and therefore the impedance of each forthcoming tissue can be determined.

Once the location of each interface is known and the impedance values of the tissues on either side of each interface is also known, an image can be constructed. Because we are considering only the area imaged by a single sound wave, our resulting image will consist of a one-dimensional "strip" of data. Throughout this strip, the distance to each interface will of course translate into a distance along the

30

representative image. The magnitude of the impedance mismatch at each interface can be directly graphed (a format known as A-mode) but is more commonly translated to a brightness level in the image (B-mode). The sample data acquired above represents a one-dimensional region of tissue and therefore produces a one-dimensional image, as shown:

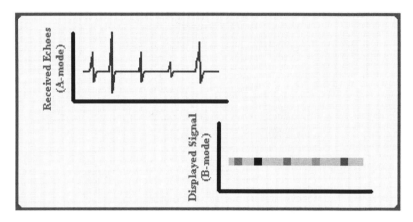

MULTIPLE LINE RECONSTRUCTION

The algorithm used in single-line reconstruction forms the backbone of ultrasound imaging; a two-dimensional image can easily be reconstructed by repeating many times the procedure for reconstructing a single line. Beginning on one edge of the area of interest, the transducer is swept across the region, acquiring one-dimensional images as described above at set spatial intervals. If each line of data is taken close enough to its adjacent line, then a complete image will be formed.

Two constraints should be noted. First, one entire line of data must be acquired before the next can be initiated. This is due to the fact that the same transducer is used for both generating the transmitted pulse and receiving the reflected echoes. Second, the entire image must be acquired and updated quickly enough that it can be perceived in real-time. The human eye works at a "speed" of 30 frames per second, therefore the entire ultrasound image must be acquired in 1/30 sec, or about 30ms. These two constraints limit how much information can be acquired since ultimately sound only travels so fast. Using a whole row of transducers rather than one transducer that repositions itself will speed up the acquisition to a large degree, but this adds physical as well as computational complexity. The temporal limitation on the depth and number of lines that can be received therefore limits the quality or resolution of the formed image.

Another geometry for acquiring multiple lines of data is the sector scan. In this format, a single transducer is again used but rather than moving it along an edge to acquire each new line, it is pivoted about a single point. This results in the familiar pie-shaped image that is most commonly seen in ultrasound. Mechanically the sector scan is much more precise and reliable than the linear-array scan.

CALCULATIONS

The first calculation that must be performed in constructing an image from received ultrasonic data is converting the amount of time to the reception of an echo pulse into the distance from the transducer to the interface that generated that pulse. The key to this relationship is acoustic velocity, which is a constant rate of distance over time. By rearranging terms, we get:

$$\text{Distance} = \text{velocity} \times \text{time}$$

In our case, the sound wave pulse must travel to the interface, then upon reflection travel back to the transducer before it is received. Thus, the distance covered is actually *twice* the actual distance between the transducer and the interface, so the more correct equation defining distance to transducer would be:

$$\text{Distance} = \tfrac{1}{2} \times \text{velocity} \times \text{time}$$

In using this relationship, we must assume that acoustic velocity remains constant. In fact, there may be minor differences in the speed of sound through various tissue types, however they are taken to be small enough to assume an average for soft tissue, 1540 m/s, as a general value. The one exception for this is the acoustic velocity of *air*, which is much lower than that of soft tissue. Special calculations may need to be made when imaging the lung or any region containing air bubbles. Once distance to the transducer has been calculated, this value is converted into a distance across the visible screen by means highly specific to the image display device.

Sound Detection/Image Formation

SWEPT GAIN CONTROL

As sound travels through a uniform medium, it does not maintain a constant intensity but is attenuated at a constant rate. This property must be taken into account when reconstructing an ultrasound image. This is again a simple calculation based on assumed known properties of the medium: given an average attenuation coefficient, the received pulses can be "regrown" or amplified to their proper intensity based on their distance from the transducer (which has already been determined.) Since amplification per distance is a constant function, the visual appearance of the correction factor is a ramp function that realigns the received pulses, such that echoes from interfaces that are farther away are amplified by a greater amount. This is sometimes referred to as swept-gain control, or time-gain control.

MECHANISMS OF RECEPTION

A transducer element converts a received ultrasound signal into an electrical stimulus; the means by which it does this is simply the reverse of how it generates sound from electronic input. In this case, the piezoelectric crystals respond to a mechanical deformation caused by sound by producing an electrical current. The magnitude of this output is proportional to the degree of deformation of the crystal, which translates to the amount of oscillation in pressure or the intensity of the incoming sound. The greater the sound wave, the greater the electrical output.

Since ultrasound signals are usually transmitted and received in pulse-mode, the process is simplified in that the transducer receives separate, discrete pulses of data rather than a continuous stream of information. Each echo pulse is separable and can be stored digitally in both the time and magnitude domains, that is the signal can be represented by a sequence of discrete values. Once the sound wave has been converted into this digital signal, it can be computationally analyzed, stored, and otherwise processed by computer in order to ultimately produce an image.

Applications and Techniques

IMPLEMENTATION

With the underlying principles in place, the next step in the development of ultrasound is to put together a device to implement these ideas. As will be explained below, an ultrasound machine contains four basic parts: a pulser, a receiver, a memory/processing unit, and a display. These parts work together to generate the transmitted sound wave pulse, receive the echoes returning from the medium, calculate from these echoes the underlying tissue structure, and display a graphical representation of this structure to the user. This process repeats itself to continuously update in real time, while a console serves as a means of adapting the device to the specific needs of the user for a given application and affects all four parts.

The job of the _pulser_ is to generate discrete electrical impulse signals at a fixed rate, each of which causes the transducer to generate an ultrasound pulse. The pulser controls both the rate at which electrical and therefore ultrasound pulses are generated (the pulse repetition frequency, or prf) and the magnitude of these pulses. Like the prf, the magnitude of the ultrasound pulses is directly proportional to the magnitude of the pulser's output signal. Larger magnitude ultrasound pulses allow greater sensitivity (that is they allow fractionally smaller echo signals to be detected) but must not exceed certain limits for safety reasons.

During the "quiet" time in between pulses being generated, the ultrasound machine "listens" for echoes returning to the transducer. This is done by the _receiver_, which accepts electrical pulses directly from the transducer and performs several preprocessing functions before passing the signal on to the central memory/processing unit:

1. _Amplification_ - Because the initial transmitted pulse is subjected to a large amount of attenuation before eventually returning to the transducer, the magnitudes of the received echoes are generally very small. In order to be interpreted as a more manageable signal to be mapped to a visible brightness range the echoes are amplified. The ratio of amplification, a constant by which the input signal is multiplied, is referred to as the gain of the receiver and is usually expressed in dB.
2. _Compensation_ - The degree of attenuation of the transmitted signal is a function of distance, therefore echoes generated by elements that are farther away from the transducer must be amplified to a greater degree than echoes generated by closer elements in order to restore each to their proper magnitude. Compensation is the application of swept-gain control to perform this correction.

34

3. Compression - Again considering the effects of attenuation, the high amount of signal loss that could occur depending on the position of the sound wave reflectors, causes a large amount of variation in the range of received echo pulses. That is in one case all of the received echoes could be of similar magnitude, while in the next case they could all be of very different magnitude. This necessitates compression, which is the standardization of the difference between the maximum and minimum received amplitudes, also called the dynamic range. Many different formulas exist for shrinking the dynamic range, such as a linear division or a logarithmic compression, in which the log of the magnitude of each echo is used. Conversely, the dynamic range could be expanded by using an exponential expansion.

4. Filtering - This process takes advantage of the fact that the ultrasound pulses that are transmitted, and therefore the echo pulses that are received, contain signals of specific, known frequency content. The receiver can eliminate unwanted noise by removing any information that is not contained within the correct frequency range and therefore improve the quality and accuracy of the signal.

5. Rejection - Another means of removing unwanted signals that do not originate from known sources, rejection is simply the process of eliminating any pulses whose magnitude falls below a certain threshold. While this may cause some "good" data to be lost, the more dominant effect is decreased noise.

6. Demodulation - A type of transduction that converts the voltage signal representing echoes to a signal in another format more appropriate for display, such as video. This signal is then passed to the memory/processing unit.

As the memory/processing unit accepts the end signal from the receiver, its task is to convert the continuous data stream into freezable images, or "frames," which are constantly updated in real time. Recall that the echo pulses at the receiver represent the interfaces of a two-dimensional space mapped to a one-dimensional, time-dependent signal. The means of mapping are based on information such as the layout of the scan lines (linear or sector), the space between scan lines, and the depth of each scan line. The memory/processing unit must deconstruct this data - it must map the sequence of echoes back to a two-dimensional image. This process is referred to as "digital scan conversion," as each scan line in digital format is converted into a section of a viewable image to be displayed. A basic visualization of this procedure for a linear scan can be formed by a checkerboard-type grid whose boxes need to be filled in. Each "box" contains data and is referred to as a pixel, which effectively represents a square region of imaged tissue. The memory/processing unit is given a sequence of digital values representing echo magnitudes and correctly maps them to the two-dimensional grid, most commonly by sweeping across horizontally, filling in pixel value brightnesses by echo magnitudes, and then moving down to the next line. For sector scans, the geometry is slightly different but the principle of image reconstruction remains the same.

The "memory" aspect of this unit involves the division of the data stream into frames. Each frame represents a single "pass" through the imaged field and is quantified by a set length of time on the data stream. The memory unit is so named because it serves the purpose of freezing each entire image while the next one is being constructed. Therefore, an entire grid of values forming an image is updated at once as new pixel values enter the data stream. When this update occurs fast enough to show instantaneous changes in the object being imaged, it is said to be in "real-time."

Any manipulation of data that occurs after the complete image is stored into the memory unit is called post-processing. The most important manipulation that is performed is assigning a brightness level to each digital value stored at the pixel locations. Other post-processing algorithms can be implemented depending on the data that is received.

Finally, the image information stored in memory is useless unless it can be visualized; this is carried out by the display. A wide range of devices can serve as a display - television, computer monitor, digital or analog. The only requirement is that it allow variable brightness levels at each pixel location in order to form an image from memory while updating rapidly enough to maintain real-time motion.

These four components - pulser, receiver, memory/processing unit, and display - work together to form the core of the ultrasound machine. The use of an ultrasound machine to perform diagnostic scans is a complex procedure that is aided by an understanding of each of these components, but nevertheless requires years of clinical experience.

DOPPLER

Doppler is a specialized application of ultrasound used to image areas that move continuously, or flow. Within the body, this specifically pertains to blood circulating throughout the vasculature. The principle behind Doppler is that for a source that provides an acoustic output of set frequency and a receiver that listens to this output, if either the source or the output is set in motion the frequency at the receiver will change. The basis of this change in frequency is an elongation or shrinking in the time domain of the transmitted sound wave as its source and receiver move away from or towards each other. Each point along its oscillation is set in motion creating a new frequency. In the example on the left the source moves from point A to point B, while in the example on the right the receiver moves from point A to point B. In both cases a "Doppler shift" will occur, the same principle by which radar waves are used by law enforcement officers to obtain vehicle speeds.

In ultrasound, the physical setup of Doppler imaging is the same as in standard ultrasound: a sound wave is transmitted by a source, reflected off of a target, then received back at the source (note that the same physical device, the transducer, acts as both source and receiver.) Because the target is a moving fluid such as blood, the reflected beam effectively comes from a moving source, and it is perceived back at the transducer as having changed in frequency.

A familiar example will confirm this result: when driving a car through a heavy rainstorm, the faster you drive the more quickly the raindrops will appear to come at you. However, in reality they are still falling at the same rate, it is the moving reference point that causes their approach, or "frequency," to change. This is essentially the same as the Doppler effect in which the source (raindrops) is stationary in relation to a moving receiver (car). As an acoustic example, consider the noise of a plane approaching overhead and then flying by. Although the sound emitted by the plane is of a set frequency, its pitch - which is related to frequency - changes as the plane flies by due to the fact that your ears represent a stationary receiver to a moving source.

No matter what the application, the Doppler effect requires a source and a target, at least one of which moves in relation to each other. Ultrasound devices are able to harness the Doppler effect to create a device that uses this frequency change to determine information about blood flow; the difference between the frequency of the transmitted signal and the frequency of the received signal is called the Doppler frequency and is used to calculate the velocity and direction of the blood flow relative to the transducer.

The basic setup for using a Doppler shift to calculate reflector velocity is as shown. A sound beam is transmitted at frequency f_o from the transducer, which reflects off of the moving fluid. The reflectors therefore act as a source that transmits a reflected beam at the same frequency f_o, but since they are in motion the perceived frequency at the transducer is a different frequency f_r. The Doppler frequency f_d is defined as the difference between these two. Clearly when the fluid is moving away from the transducer as in this case, the received frequency f_r will be less than f_o, the velocity of the reflectors is in a sense "subtracted" from the velocity of the oscillations of the sound wave.

$$f_d = f_o - f_r$$

Next, this Doppler frequency is used to calculate the velocity of the moving fluid by another equation that defines Doppler frequency in terms of initial frequency, reflector velocity (V) and the speed of sound (c):

$$v = \frac{(f_d \times c)}{2f_o}$$

Hardware Controls

While the layout and appearance of ultrasound devices can vary based on manufacturer and model, several universal console elements allow control over the most common processes and settings. The first and most important setting is transducer frequency, which affects a number of characteristics of the image acquisition including beam formation, scatter, and attenuation. Since each piezoelectric element has its own operating frequency, a different physical transducer must be used for each desired beam frequency. Another common feature, pulse repetition frequency, is more readily adjustable by simply altering the rate of electrical stimuli to the pulser; this value is adjusted in order to change the maximum depth that can be imaged.

Turning our attention closer to the signal, the properties of the individual pulse waveforms can be adjusted in order to improve axial resolution. As the duration of the pulse is increased, a larger (worse) axial resolution results. Since each pulse generated by the transducer is a result of a single stimulus from the pulser, the system has no direct means of controlling pulse duration other than changing the physics of the transducer element. Instead, pulse duration is controlled by the amount of damping applied to the pulse after generation. Damping is caused by backing material and/or matching layers and so it is these elements that are influenced by console elements governing pulse duration.

Adjustment of swept-gain is vital to producing an accurate image. The actual controls usually consist of a set of sliding knobs, each mapped to a set distance. The standard setting would be linear, that is greater distances receiving greater amplification, however other layouts may prove more effective after a trial-and-error adjustment period. For example, the existence of bone at a certain depth would cause a large amount of attenuation, therefore the region past it would require greater amplification. Most commonly, the barrier between the imaged tissue and the exterior causes a disruption in the linear attenuation slope.

The display unit has a number of controls that act independently of the image acquisition process but nonetheless affect the end result. These are dependent on the unit and include common settings such as brightness, contrast, etc.

Many other processing algorithms can be put under control of the user. Some of the more standard ones have already been mentioned - rejection, compression (logarithmic vs. linear) - while many others have recently been or are being developed. Each machine and each manufacturer will implement its own preprocessing and postprocessing algorithms, some specific to a given application, to create what the designers believe to be the most detailed and most accurate image.

COUPLING GEL

One of the first things you'll notice as a patient if you have an ultrasound performed is the application of coupling gel around the area being imaged. The reason this gel is required comes down to the fundamental properties of sound propagation that we have studied: recall that reflection of the sound occurs at impedance boundaries and is a function of the difference in impedance on either side of these boundaries. Also recall that air is a medium having one of the lowest impedances to sound. Putting these two pieces of information together, it is clear that if the face of the transducer that generates the sound wave does not make continuous contact with the skin that overlays the bodily tissue to be imaged, the impending air-tissue interface will preclude any sound propagation from occurring through the body.

The purpose of the coupling gel, therefore, is to remove the air boundary and to allow the transducer-skin interface to maintain as constant an impedance as possible, thus preventing reflection from occurring in this region. The impedance of the coupling gel should be as close as possible to that of the skin surface. Also note that the inner workings of the transducer itself must contain a matching layer such that as sound is generated from its piezoelectric crystal and propagated out its face, the impedance of the material through which it flows matches that of the coupling gel and the bodily tissue.

NEW MODES

A rapidly developing innovation in ultrasound imaging is that of three-dimensional ultrasound. This process uses a variety of different techniques to acquire a visualized projection of a 3-D volume onto a 2-D image, allowing more information and detail than a standard two-dimensional linear or sector scan. The process of obtaining this volume of data is an extension of the same principles used in 2-D ultrasound with the added steps of sending and receiving sound pulses in multiple planes. Each time this is done, the system must recognize the location of the transducer and direction of the sound beam in order to reconstruct the 3-D volume. The exact physics of how this is done depends on the particular system and application. Because this process takes more time than a 2-D acquisition, movement of the patient becomes an issue, and real-time updates are more difficult to achieve. Various coding or compressional techniques may need to be used.

Contrast agents are used in ultrasound in a fashion similar to those used in radiology. The agent is injected into the bloodstream prior to an image acquisition. When viewing the resulting ultrasound image, the contrast agent stands out against its background, therefore emphasizing the bloodstream and vasculature. This process is frequently used in cardiology in order to image the heart. For the purpose of ultrasound, the contrast agent must have a high reflection coefficient in order to stand out in the image. As we know, air presents the highest impedance mismatch to soft tissue. Therefore, ultrasound contrast agents typically utilize microscopic air bubbles to produce a fluid that reflects sound to a high degree and will be easily visible within the acquired image. Of course, the agent must also be safe for the patient and be cleared from the body in due time.

Another new development in ultrasound is known as Native Tissue Harmonic Imaging (NTHI). To summarize, the property that is utilized in NTHI is the fact that when directing an ultrasound beam into the body, the echoes that return have components not only at the fundamental frequency of the transmitted beam, as previously described, but also at frequencies of integer multiples of this fundamental frequency. For example, if a 2MHz sound wave is transmitted into the body, echoes will return to the transducer having components at frequencies of 2MHz, 4MHz, 6MHz, 8MHz, etc. (These integer multiples are known as the harmonic frequencies in this case). The reason for these harmonic-frequency components is the change in acoustic velocity that occurs as the propagating medium is alternately compressed and relaxed by the sound wave. At each increasing harmonic frequency, the magnitude of the corresponding component of the received echo decreases in magnitude: the majority of information will be contained at the fundamental frequency, the first harmonic (at 4MHz in the example above) will have a lower magnitude, the second harmonic will have a lower magnitude still, and so forth. When transmitting and receiving an ultrasound wave, a large portion of the artifacts/noise that are present are caused by the exterior body wall and are carried only at the fundamental frequency. Therefore, the process of NTHI involves filtering the received echo signal in such a manner as to remove the components that are at the fundamental frequency, leaving only the components at the harmonic frequencies. The result is an improved signal-to-noise ratio and a sharper image.

SAFETY

As in all imaging procedures, safety to the patient and to the operator are of primary concern. A major benefit of ultrasound is its lack of damaging energy common to x-ray-based modalities. For this reason, ultrasound is the imaging technique of choice for fetal imaging. Of course, ultrasound waves of sufficient magnitude and/or frequency would be capable of causing damage to body tissue, therefore the operation of ultrasound devices must be governed by predetermined acceptable limits. Clinical trials to determine these levels have been somewhat inconclusive. The impact of sound waves on tissue appear to be largely dependent on the particular tissue being imaged. Nevertheless, all data does support that waves of less than $100mW/cm^2$ have no damaging bioeffects and are therefore considered safe.

A secondary effect of the transmission of ultrasonic waves into the body is known as cavitation. A rapid decrease in surrounding pressure induced by the sound wave causes bubbles in the medium to expand; subsequent increase in surrounding pressure causes the same bubbles to collapse as well as to increase in internal pressure and in temperature. This increase in temperature may cause serious biological effects, to say nothing of the damaging effects of air bubbles on the quality of the acquired ultrasound image. This process is known as transient cavitation and occurs at high sound wave intensities. At lower intensities, stable cavitation occurs; here the bubbles do not completely collapse. Cavitation can be minimized by removing gas from the imaged medium, by applying external pressure to the

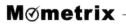

medium, by using a higher frequency sound wave, or most simply by using a lower intensity sound wave.

Image Features

The fundamental principles that underlie the generation of an ultrasound image are well defined and under ideal circumstances will allow an exact image representation of a solid medium with perfect features. When applied to the human body, which is extremely non-ideal, many of these fundamentals break down, or at least begin to behave in an unanticipated manner, resulting in an image whose features contain artifacts that must be interpreted properly to gain a correct evaluation of the imaged tissue. By understanding how these fundamentals act imperfectly and recognizing common image features and artifacts, a more correct evaluation can be made.

SCATTERERS

The most noticeable feature of displayed ultrasound images is the fuzzy or grainy texture about the entire image. This is due to a process known as scatter, which was introduced in section 2. Because each scatterer is small relative to the tissue being imaged, the propagating sound wave as a whole remains intact, however scatterers do account for a decrease in image quality: at impedance boundaries they cause blurring and decreased intensity while within the medium they create speckle. Even though the presence of scatterers in ultrasound must be accepted, their effect on image quality can be managed to some degree by adjusting properties such as transducer frequency; as explained in section 2 a lower frequency will be less subject to the effects of scattering. However, this must be weighed against the many other features that affect image quality.

SHADOWING/ENHANCEMENT

Almost all ultrasound devices include a swept-gain control function, as described in section 3. Assuming these controls to be properly calibrated, the displayed image corresponding to a given area of the body should be of uniform intensity, or brightness, across all depths. In practice, however, it is almost impossible to perfectly calibrate the swept-gain control; the result is one of two artifacts: shadowing and enhancement. A "shadow" is cast by any imaged tissue whose rate of attenuation of sound is greater than that of the background, surrounding medium. The added loss in intensity as sound propagates through this portion of the medium will mean that attenuation will be greater than the amount that is accounted for by the SGC. As a result, the transmitted sound beam at all points beyond this tissue will be of lower intensity than what is expected, and the image corresponding to those points will be of lower brightness than expected.

The most logical means of accounting for this extraordinary loss of sonic magnitude would be to fine-tune the swept-gain control such that the lost intensity is "added back" to the signal at the proper depth. This would require an advanced knowledge of the region being imaged, would not be very accurate, and would introduce additional noise and other artifacts into the image. Instead, consider the influence of frequency on the degree of shadowing. Like almost every aspect of ultrasound,

sound wave frequency has a pronounced effect on shadowing and must be selected carefully to maintain a delicate balance of all dependent factors. Because higher frequency sound waves are subject to a higher rate of attenuation, they are also corrected to a higher degree by the SGC, that is the controls form a "steeper" angle. So, when propagating through a high-attenuating material, the degree of shadowing that results after correction also becomes greater. Because the high-attenuating material is of a fixed width, a greater amount of signal loss that is not completely corrected for by the SGC will occur across this width.

The opposite effect of shadowing can occur by the same principle: if a part of the imaged medium has a rate of attenuation that is lower than that of the surrounding medium, there will be less of a loss in intensity than was originally accounted for. As a result, all points beyond along the axis of the sound beam will have a higher sound wave intensity and higher projected image brightness level than the baseline, a phenomenon known as enhancement. Like shadowing, enhancement is a function of transducer frequency and must be recognized when analyzing ultrasound images.

REVERBERATION

The transmitted and reflected sound waves discussed so far have been limited to intended signals that return necessary information. However, the tissue medium holds no discrimination for signals that are desired by the ultrasound device and other signals that propagate through; all behave the same way. A significant artifact that can result from unintended sound waves is reverberation. To explain, consider once again a simplified layout containing only the transducer placed on the surface of the skin and a single tissue (say, muscle) held within a surrounding medium (water). The desired effect is for the transmitted sound beam to reflect off of each interface and return to the transducer:

It cannot be ignored that the sound wave will *continue to propagate* and therefore continue to reflect off of each interface, i.e. it will reverberate. Upon returning to the transducer, the sound wave will reflect back at the medium and again undergo its original path. As you can see, this will eventually cause the transducer to receive a signal that corresponds to a location beyond the farthest edge of the tissue layout.

While this incorrect information can be removed by simply limiting the displayed image to a specified depth (either temporally or spatially), similar artifacts can always occur due to reverberation between any two interfaces. Consider the situation below:

The sound wave will continue to "bounce" between the interfaces at A and B, each time returning part of its signal back to the transducer. Because both interfaces are close to the transducer, the reverberation artifacts appear within the limits of the image, and will continue until the sound wave magnitude is attenuated below a minimum level. There is no real solution to reverberation, other than being aware of its presence and learning to identify situations where it is likely to occur.

DEFLECTION

As described in section 2, refraction occurs whenever an incident sound beam strikes an interface at a non-perpendicular angle. What must also be accounted for is the deflective effect that this has on regeneration of the image. As can be seen below, a transmitted beam that refracts at an interface, strikes a reflecting interface, then refracts back towards the transducer on return will be received and interpreted as being positioned along a straight axis from the transducer. The system can only assume that sound travels in a straight line away from and then back towards the transducer, although when refraction occurs this is not the actual case. The end result is improper positioning of interfaces on the final image.

RESOLUTION

The resolution of an image is perceived as the sharpness or quality of the image; it is a function of the number of pixels in the image, or the size of each of these pixels. A given physiological region can theoretically be imaged at any resolution, depending on the properties of the imaging equipment. Mathematically, resolution is the smallest possible distance between two points on the image such that the two points can still be distinguished from each other. A higher resolution is preferred, this means the viewer can separate two points that are very close to each other; the image contains more information and is visually more detailed. Note that the designation "high resolution" implies "better" resolution, which actually corresponds to resolution having a lower numerical value and smaller pixel size.

The size of a square pixel is of course based on its two dimensions, width and height. In ultrasound terms, the width and height axes correspond to a distance and rotation from the transducer origin, while resolution is expressed in terms of these two lengths. Distance from the transducer is referred to as range while rotation from the main axis is referred to as azimuth; both are usually measured in mm. The resolution in these two dimensions in ultrasound is constrained by properties of the transmitted sound wave that is used and by the setup of the ultrasound machine.

Range resolution is limited by the duration of each transmitted sound pulse. Each pulse propagates away from transducer, along the range axis. Two objects that are close enough to each other relative to the duration of the transmitted pulse will be interpreted as one single, larger object and will be indistinguishable from each other in the final image. Pulse duration is another property that is affected by the transducer frequency setting.

Azimuth resolution is limited by beam width. Two objects whose distance between each other is smaller than the width of the sound beam will similarly be grouped together and imaged as a single object. As previously described, beam width is determined by the physical dimensions of the transducer element and is adjustable to some extent. The narrowest part of the beam, and therefore the highest resolution, occurs in the focal region.

These absolute resolution limits are defined by the sound beam, but in ultrasound practice the more applicable resolution limits are set by the constraints of real-time updating. Recall that the entire displayed ultrasound image must be continuously reacquired and redrawn at a rate fast enough that motion is perceived by the viewer. The human eye updates at 30 fps, so each two-dimensional image must be acquired in 1/30 sec or about 33ms. Since the amount of time available for acquiring an image is limited, resolution ultimately comes down to the speed of sound, which cannot be altered. Given this fixed amount of time to work with during which the sound wave must be transmitted and received at each image line, there is a tradeoff that must be made between the number of imaged lines within the region in question (azimuth resolution) and the depth of each imaged line. First a maximum depth from the transducer that the image must cover is selected; from this value the number of lines that can be scanned within 33ms is calculated and these lines are evenly spaced throughout the imaged region, setting the azimuth resolution.

Resolution describes the degree of image definition not only in the two spatial dimensions but also in the intensity dimension. In a similar manner as with spatial resolution, intensity resolution is quantified by the smallest possible detectable change in intensity between two points. Since the image is stored digitally, the number of possible values that a pixel may have or number of bits of storage at each pixel makes up the image intensity resolution. Intensity resolution can be improved by increasing the magnitude of the transmitted sound wave, allowing smaller fractional changes in received pulses to be detected. Intensity resolution is also limited by the storage space and speed of the ultrasound device that processes all of the information.

ULTRASOUND VS. SOUND IN NORMAL HEARING RANGE

Characteristic	Sound in normal hearing range	Ultrasound
Frequency	20 Hz – 20 kHz	Over 20 kHz For medical imaging, 1 MHz – 15 MHz
Audibility	Audible to humans	Inaudible to humans
Wavelength	Longer wavelength	Shorter wavelength
Scattering	More easily scattered	Less easily scattered by body tissue

PIEZOELECTRIC EFFECT VS. ALTERNATING POTENTIAL EFFECT

- Certain crystalline materials, with fixed ions in the crystalline lattice, exhibit an effect in which mechanical stress applied to the crystal produces a potential difference between opposite faces. This effect is called the piezoelectric effect.

- Conversely, a potential difference applied to opposite faces of the crystal, say by two electrodes on either side of a flat slab of piezoelectric crystal, causes mechanical deformation of the crystal. If an alternating potential difference is applied, the crystal vibrates, that is, becomes alternately thinner then fatter between the electrodes, at the same the frequency as the applied potential difference.
- If the vibrating crystal is in contact with air, it will produce a sound wave of the same frequency as the alternating potential difference. The frequency of the applied alternating potential difference is chosen to give the desired frequency of ultrasound. Careful sizing of the crystal material, to match its natural resonant vibration to this frequency, makes for the most efficient transfer of electrical energy to ultrasound energy.

ACOUSTIC IMPEDANCE

- **Acoustic impedance**, Z, is the opposition of a medium to the passage of sound waves. A substance with a high acoustic impedance hinders the movement of sound energy more than a substance with a low acoustic impedance.
- Impedance is proportional to both the density of the medium and the velocity of the sound within it. The units for acoustic impedance can be found by multiplying the units for density by the units for velocity. Hence, acoustic impedance is measured in $kgm^{-2}s^{-1}$.
- The body consists of a range of materials, such as air in the lungs, gas in the bowel, water, blood, muscle, fat and bone. Each body component has a characteristic impedance that depends upon the nature of the matter in it. Gases have very low density, therefore very low acoustic impedance. The impedance of a particular tissue will vary within a range around a typical value.

Substance	Characteristic acoustic impedance
Air	$429 \ kgm^{-2}s^{-1}$
Water	$1.43 \times 10^6 \ kgm^{-2}s^{-1}$

SAMPLE CALCULATION

The density of blood is $1060 \ kgm^{-3}$ and its ultrasound velocity is $1570 \ ms^{-1}$

Acoustic impedance, $Z = \rho v = 1060 \times 1570 = 1.59 \times 10^6 \ kgm^{-2}s^{-1}$

Ultrasound will move through a medium until it encounters a boundary. When this happens, some ultrasounds will be reflected from the boundary and some will cross the boundary. The ratio of these two amounts depends upon the difference between their acoustic impedance. A big difference will mean that very little of the sound will cross the boundary. This means that the boundary will give a strong echo.
Ultrasound echoes are the basis of examining tissues. Bone has the highest acoustic impedance in the body and so most sound is reflected from the surface of the bone.

This means that the sound cannot penetrate the bone. Tissues enclosed by bone, (eg in the skull) hidden by bone or within bone cannot be examined.

For a similar reason air interfaces have almost complete reflection. This means that tissues with enclosed air, such as the lungs, are difficult to image.

On the other hand, adjacent tissues with similar acoustic impedances will allow some ultrasound to be transmitted and some reflected. This allows both an echo and further penetration of the ultrasound. Each boundary will give an echo a short time later than the preceding one. This allows us to examine the tissue the sound has just passed through. Thus, soft or watery tissues such as muscle, fat and blood can be examined.

PRINCIPLES OF ACOUSTIC IMPEDANCE AND REFLECTION AND REFRACTION APPLIED TO ULTRASOUND

- A short burst (pulse) of ultrasound is produced by a piezoelectric transducer. This pulse will travel through a medium until it reaches the boundary with another medium.
- Some of the pulse will be reflected and will return to the transducer. The distance from the transducer to the boundary (ie the depth of the boundary) can be found by recording the time between the pulse and its echo.
- Some of the pulse will cross the boundary (ie be refracted) into the second medium. This refracted pulse will continue into the second medium until it reaches another boundary, where some of it will be reflected to return to the transducer and some will be refracted a second time. In this way a series of echoes having different time lags from the initial burst will be recorded. Each represents a boundary at a different distance (depth) from the transducer.
- The amount of ultrasound reflected compared to the amount refracted at a boundary will depend upon the different acoustic impedances of each medium. A large difference in impedance means that there is more reflection and less refraction at a boundary.

The **A scan** consists of a series of amplitude peaks on a cathode ray oscilloscope (CRO) trace, each peak corresponding to an echo from a boundary of a certain depth. The CRO trace is actually a time scale but knowing the pulse velocity allows us to determine distance, that is, the depth of the boundary that returned an echo. **A scans** are used in situations where only distance measurements are required. Two such situations are measurements in the eye and foetal skull size. The latter can be used to estimate the developmental stage of the foetus. **A scans** require less complex equipment than other ultrasound techniques.

B SCANS

- B (brightness) scans show the echo as a brightness signal on the CRO.
- A static **B scan** consists of a series of bright dots.
- Each dot on a static **B scan** corresponds to an echo from a boundary of a certain depth.

- Static **B scans** are not very useful on their own
- **B scans** form the basis of sector and phase scans.

EXAMPLE OF A TABLE

Scan type	Description	Example of use	Reason for use
Phase scan	The ultrasound probe has many transducers. These are arranged to send pulses at slightly different times, that is, with a different phase. In this way the overall wavefront will travel in a certain direction. This allows the pulse to be directed in a sweep to build up a cross sectional image.	obstetrics abdominal investigations cardiography	shows a two-dimensional image produces good image quality
Sector scan	Successive B scans are made as the transducer probe is rocked sideways on the patient. Each static B scan is added to form a fan-shaped (sector) brightness image. This is a cross-sectional image.	imaging of the infant brain through the fontanel	shows a two-dimensional image only needs a small entry 'window'.

USE OF DOPPLER EFFECT IN ULTRASONICS TO OBTAIN FLOW CHARACTERISTICS OF BLOOD MOVING THROUGH THE HEART

- The **Doppler effect** is the apparent change in wavelength of a wave when it is produced by a source moving relative to a stationary observer. When a source of sound waves moves towards an observer, the waves are 'bunched up'; their wavelength is shorter and the frequency heard by the observer is higher. The converse is true when the source is moving away from the observer. The Doppler effect also happens if the source is stationary and the observer is moving.
- If a pulse of ultrasound reflects off a stationary boundary it will return with the same frequency and wavelength as was emitted. If the boundary is moving away from the transducer there will be a Doppler shift effect. The waves will undergo a Doppler shift on their outward and reflected journeys, producing a double Doppler shift.
- Ultrasound used in blood flow measurement is typically in the range 5 to 15 MHz. The 'moving boundary' comprises the surfaces of multiple red blood cells, as an individual red blood cell is too small to be a boundary on its own. The Doppler shift is typically a change in frequency of up to 3 kHz. This value is positive when blood flows towards the probe, and negative when the blood flows away.

- Sophisticated computer software can assign colours to an ultrasound scan on the basis of its Doppler shift. In this way flow velocity can be seen. A colour change can indicate increased velocity, indicating a narrowed artery. Colour intensity can indicate flow volume. Mixed colours can indicate flow turbulence due to a partial blockage. The wrong colour can indicate a leaking heart valve. Doppler shifts can be in the audible range and so can be heard. An experienced operator can make a diagnosis using this sound.

The ratio of reflected to initial intensity as: $\frac{I_r}{I_o} = \frac{[Z_2 - Z_1]^2}{[Z_2 + Z_1]^2}$

- You should be able to clearly indicate that 'intensity' is a measure of the energy in the pulse of ultrasound and that it depends upon the amplitude of the waves in a pulse of a certain frequency. You should also be able to indicate that acoustic impedance is a function of the density of a material and the velocity of the waves in that material.

Resolution, Beamforming and the Point Spread Function

A typical transducer uses an array of piezoelectric elements to transmit a sound pulse into the body and to receive the echoes that return from scattering structures within. This array is often referred to as the imaging system's **aperture**. The transmit signals passing to, and the received signals passing from the array elements can be individually delayed in time, hence the term **phased array**. This is done to electronically steer and focus each of a sequence of acoustic pulses through the plane or volume to be imaged in the body. This produces a 2- or 3-D map of the scattered echoes, or **tissue echogenicity** that is presented to the clinician for interpretation. The process of steering and focusing these acoustic pulses is known as **beamforming**. This process is shown schematically in Figure 1.1.

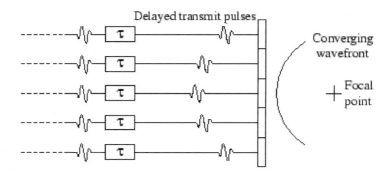

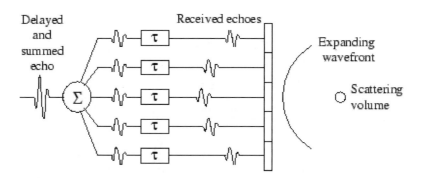

Figure 1.1: A conceptual diagram of phased array beamforming. (Top) Appropriately delayed pulses are transmitted from an array of piezoelectric elements to achieve steering and focusing at the point of interest. (For simplicity, only focusing delays are shown here.) (Bottom) The echoes returning are likewise delayed before they are summed together to form a strong echo signal from the region of interest.

50

The ability of a particular ultrasound system to discriminate closely spaced scatterers is specified by its spatial resolution, which is typically defined as the minimum scatterer spacing at which this discrimination is possible. The system resolution has three components in Cartesian space, reflecting the spatial extent of the ultrasound pulse at the focus. The coordinates of this space are in the axial, lateral, and elevation dimensions. The axial, or **range**, dimension indicates the predominant direction of sound propagation, extending from the transducer into the body. The axial and the lateral dimension together define the tomographic plane, or slice, of the displayed image. These dimensions relative to the face of a linear array transducer are shown in Figure 1.2. The elevation dimension contains the slice thickness.

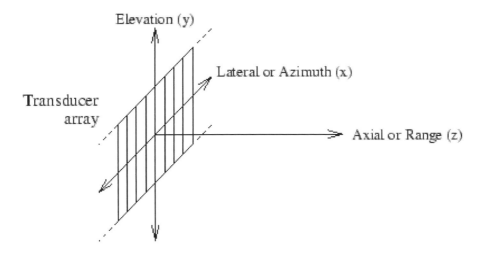

Figure 1.2: A diagram of the spatial coordinate system used to describe the field and resolution of an ultrasound transducer array. Here the transducer is a 1-D array, subdivided into elements in the lateral dimension. The transmitted sound pulse travels out in the axial dimension.

A modern ultrasound scanner operating in brightness mode, or **B-mode**, presents the viewer with a gray-scale image that represents a map of echo amplitude, or **brightness,** as a function of position in the region being scanned. In B-mode the ultrasound system interrogates the region of interest with wide bandwidth sound pulses. Such a pulse from a typical array is shown in Figure 1.3.

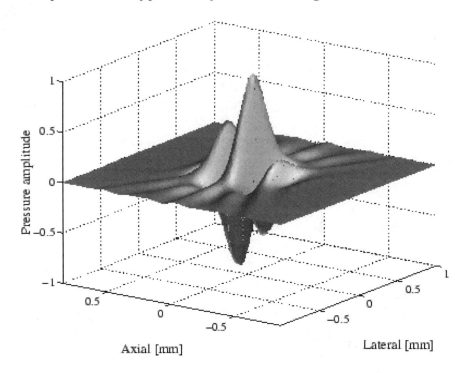

Figure 1.3: The acoustic pulse from a typical array (7.5 MHz, 60% bandwidth, 128 elements of width equal to the wavelength), shown at the acoustic focus. The pulse is displayed as a map of pressure amplitude and is traveling in the positive direction along axial dimension.

The acoustic pulse in Figure 1.3 is shown as a function of acoustic pressure over the lateral and axial dimensions. In fact, the pulse is a three-dimensional function, with extent in elevation as well. In the terminology of linear systems theory, it is the impulse response of the system, and the response of the ultrasound system at the focus is fully characterized by this function. As it represents the output of the ultrasound system during interrogation of an ideal point target, it is also known as the system's **point spread function** (PSF). The character of the PSF in the axial dimension is determined predominantly by the center frequency and bandwidth of the acoustic signal generated at each transducer element, while its character in the lateral and elevation dimensions is determined predominantly by the aperture and element geometries and the beamforming applied. The term PSF is often used to refer to two-dimensional representations of the system response in pressure amplitude versus space, such as that shown in Figure 1.3, with the implicit understanding that the actual response has three-dimensional extent.

In analyzing hypothetical ultrasound systems, predicting the form of the PSF is critical. However, the analytic solution for the PSF for an arbitrary array geometry is usually intractable. Throughout this document, an acoustic field simulation program developed by Jensen and Svendsen was used to predict the acoustic field under the various conditions and array geometries of interest. This program is based on a method developed by Tupholme and Stephanishen. It calculates the convolution of a transmit excitation function, such as a sine wave with Gaussian envelope, with the spatial impulse response of the transducer. The spatial impulse response is the hypothetical pressure pattern created upon excitation of the array with a perfect impulse. The spatial impulse response is not a physically realizable, but serves as a useful calculation tool in this context. This method can accommodate arbitrary geometries by division of the aperture into smaller, rectangular elements. The spatial impulse response for each element is calculated separately, and then these solutions are combined by superposition to produce that for the entire aperture.

The **sound** in ultrasound is a physical longitudinal wave. The compression and rarefaction of the medium at the wavefront causes particle translations on the order of microns. The tissue at the cellular level is perturbed on a bulk level, i.e. the wavelength is much greater than the size of cells.

Here are some numbers of interest to put ultrasound in perspective. At 1 MHz, $100 mW/cm^2$ (FDA upper acoustic power limit):

Wavelengthmm	
Phase velocity	1540m/s = 1.54mm/µs
Peak particle displacement	0.0057µm
Peak particle velocity	3.8 cm/sec
Peak particle acceleration	22,452 g
Peak pressure	1.8 atm
Radiation force	0.007 g/cm2
Heat equivalent	0.024 cal/sec cm2 (total absorption)

The Scattering and Reflection of Sound

Medical ultrasound imaging relies utterly on the fact that biological tissues scatter or reflect incident sound. Although the phenomenon is closely related, in this text scattering refers to the interaction between sound waves and particles that are much smaller than the sound's wavelength λ, while reflection refers to such interaction with particles or objects larger than λ.

The scattering or reflection of acoustic waves arise from inhomogeneities in the medium's density and/or compressibility. Sound is primarily scattered or reflected by a discontinuity in the medium's mechanical properties, to a degree proportional to the discontinuity. (By contrast, continuous changes in a medium's material properties cause the direction of propagation to change gradually.) The elasticity and density of a material are related to its sound speed, and thus sound is scattered or reflected most strongly by significant discontinuities in the density and/or sound speed of the medium.

RAYLEIGH – TYNDALL SCATTERING

Backscattering of ultrasound from blood. The echoes detected from blood (e.g. in Doppler ultrasound) are created through interference between scattered wavelets from numerous point scatterers. The intensity of the backscattered echoes is proportional to the total number of scatterers, which means that the echo amplitude is proportional to the square root of the total number of scatterers. At normal blood flow, the number of point scatterers in blood is proportional to the number of red blood cells (i.e. the amount of blood). When blood flow is turbulent, or accelerating fast (e.g. in a stenosis), the number of inhomogeneities in the red blood cell concentration will increase, thus giving rise to stronger echoes than can be accounted for by merely the amount of blood. The intensity of the backscattered ultrasound is also proportional to the fourth power of ultrasound frequency. Doubling the ultrasonic frequency makes the echoes from blood 16 times as strong. (On the other hand, higher frequency ultrasound suffers from higher attenuation in the tissues.)

FOCUSING

In ultrasound imaging, the focusing of the ultrasound beam by means of acoustic lenses or electronic focusing. The ultrasound transmitted from the transducer crystal can be considered to be composed of multiple wavelets that interact constructively to create a wavefront (see Huygens principle). In an acoustic lens, the speed of sound is higher than in the soft tissues in front of the lens, and wavelets that have traveled the longest distance through a concave lens, i.e. the more peripheral ones, will be ahead of the more centrally located wavelets after the lens is passed. The wavefront is therefore curved, and the ultrasound beam becomes focused. A concave transducer surface would give the same effect. The principle is valid for electronic focusing as well.

ULTRASOUND BEAM

The confined, directional beam of ultrasound travelling as a longitudinal wave from the transducer face into the propagation medium. Two separate regions along the beam can be identified, the near field or Fresnel zone, and the far field or Fraunhofer zone. A confined, slightly converging beam shape is maintained in the near field owing to constructive and destructive interference patterns of individual sound wavelets emitted from the surface of the transducer crystal. The length of the near field is equal to $r^2/\lambda = d^2/4\,\lambda$, where r is the radius and d the diameter of the transducer crystal, and λ is the ultrasound wavelength in the medium of propagation. Maximum ultrasound intensity occurs at the near field - far field interface. Beam divergence in the far field results in a continuous loss of ultrasound intensity with distance from the transducer. The angle of divergence in the far field, q, is approximately equal to arcsin $(1.22\,\lambda/d)$ (or sin q = 1.22l λ/d). Note that with increasing transducer frequency (decreasing wavelength), the length of the near field increases and the angle of divergence in the far field decreases. Both changes improve lateral resolution in deep structures, but this beneficial effect of high transducer frequency is counteracted by the decrease in penetration. An increase in the diameter of the transducer crystal will also increase the length of the near field and decrease the angle of divergence, but with the drawback of a wider ultrasound beam and therefore decreased lateral resolution in the near field.

INTENSITY OF SOUND

Acoustic energy (joule) per unit time (second) and unit area (square metre). Acoustic power is acoustic energy per unit time and is measured in watts (W), 1 W being 1 joule/s. The intensity of sound is thus the acoustic power per unit area, measured in W/m^2. The intensity is determined by the amplitudes or excursions of the particles conducting the waves; the larger the amplitudes of oscillation, the higher the intensity. The actual relationship is $I = p^2/2Z$, where I is intensity, p is pressure amplitude, and Z is acoustic impedance.

SPEED OF SOUND

The propagation speed of a sound wave (e.g. ultrasound) through a medium. The propagation speed is determined by the physical properties of the medium, and is independent of the (ultra)sound frequency. The major parameters affecting the speed of sound (c) are the elasticity (K) and density (ρ) of the medium, their relationship being $c = \sqrt{(K/\rho)}$

High elasticity implies large elastic forces between the particles of the medium and a high resistance against compression (low compressibility). Speed increases with decreasing compressibility (increasing elasticity) because less compressible media have more densely packed molecules which need to move only a small distance before their motion is transmitted to the neighboring molecules. Speed decreases with increasing density because dense materials tend to have large, heavy molecules that are difficult to start and stop in the rhythmic motion involved in the propagation of sound. Tissues may be considered liquids, and in liquids, compressibility and density are generally inversely proportional. The speed of sound is therefore very similar in all tissues, the average speed in human soft tissue being approximately 1540 m/s.

LONGITUDINAL WAVE

A waveform transmitted through a medium where the particles of the medium oscillate in the direction of the wave propagation. Sound propagates as longitudinal waves. A longitudinal wave is produced when a vibrator, e.g. a piezoelectric crystal in an ultrasound transducer, transmits its back and forth oscillation into a continuous, elastic medium. The particles of the medium are made to oscillate in the direction of the wave propagation, but are otherwise stationary. The wave propagates as bands of compression and rarefaction. One wavelength is the distance between two bands of compression, or rarefaction. Maximum compression corresponds to maximum pressure.

PULSE REPETITION FREQUENCY (PRF)

In pulsed ultrasound, the number of pulses transmitted per second. For imaging, the PRF is usually in the range of 1 000 to 5 000 pulses per second, i.e. 15 kHz. The PRF is limited by the range to be examined. To avoid range ambiguity, the echoes from the deepest structures must be allowed to return to the transducer before the next pulse is transmitted. In pulsed Doppler ultrasound, the PRF determines the maximum measurable velocity.

ULTRASOUND PULSE

A short-duration wave of ultrasound. Pulses of ultrasound, as opposed to continuous wave ultrasound, are used in all ultrasound applications based on the pulse - echo method, such as A-mode, M-mode, B-mode, colour Doppler sonography, power Doppler sonography, and pulsed Doppler ultrasound. The pulse duration and spatial pulse length are determined by factors such as the Q factor of the transducer crystal and by the characteristics of the backing block of the transducer. Typically, B-mode applications use very short pulses to ensure high axial resolution, while Doppler ultrasound requires longer lasting pulses to provide a more narrow spectrum of ultrasound frequencies. There is a reciprocal relationship between the pulse duration and the pulse bandwidth (defined as width of energy spectrum at half height): pulse bandwidth (MHz) ~ 1/pulse duration (ms).

A-MODE

Amplitude mode, a one-dimensional ultrasonic display showing echoes along the ultrasonic beam as vertical spikes on a horizontal time axis indicating the depth of the reflectors. The amplitudes of the spikes reflect the echo strengths after time gain compensation TGC, and the left-right position of the spikes is determined by the time lag between transmission of the ultrasonic pulse and arrival of the echo at the transducer. The later the arrival of the echoes, the further to the right their display.

B-MODE

Brightness mode, a two-dimensional ultrasound image display composed of bright dots representing the ultrasound echoes. The brightness of each dot is determined by the echo amplitude (after time gain compensation TGC). A B-mode image is produced by sweeping a narrow ultrasound beam through the region of interest while transmitting pulses and detecting echoes along a series of closely spaced scan lines. The scanning may be performed with a single transducer mounted on an articulating arm that provides information on the ultrasound beam direction (compound B scan, static B scanner), or with a real-time scanner such as a mechanical scanner or an electronic array scanner. A linear array transducer with multiple crystal elements is used. At each scan line position, one ultrasound pulse is transmitted and all echoes from the surface to the deepest range are recorded before the ultrasound beam moves on to the next scan line position where pulse transmission and echo recording are repeated. In the B-mode image, the vertical (depth) position of each bright dot is determined by the time delay from pulse transmission to return of the echo, and the horizontal position by the location of the receiving transducer element. A shadowing artefact (distal to the bone and to the lateral edges of the fluid-filled cyst), and an enhancement artefact (distal to the cyst) are also shown.

M-Mode

Motion mode, also called time motion (TM) mode. An ultrasonic display showing A-mode data (echoes) as dots along a vertical depth axis, as opposed to the normal A-mode presentation of spikes along a horizontal depth (time) axis. The brightness of the dots is determined by the echo strength. For each pulse repetition period (PRP), a new set of vertical A-mode data is acquired and the old A-mode data are pushed to the left on the monitor to make room for the new data that are appearing on the right side of the screen. In this way, the dots are made to scroll across the screen (or alternatively on a strip of paper), thus creating bright curves indicating vertical positional changes of the reflectors with time. The M-mode curves provide very detailed information on the motional behavior of reflecting structures along the ultrasound beam and the method is especially popular in cardiology to show the motion patterns of the various cardiac valve leaflets.

The Q factor of an ultrasound transducer is defined as:

$$Q = f0 / (f2 - f1)$$

where f0 is the resonant frequency (centre frequency) of the transducer crystal, f2 is the frequency above resonance at which the intensity is reduced by half, and f1 is the frequency below resonance at which the intensity is reduced by half. f2 - f1 is thus an expression of the band width of the sound.

The Q factor refers to two characteristics of the transducer: the "purity" (bandwidth) of the sound and the persistence of the sound (the ring down time). Bandwidth and sound duration are related. Theoretically, only infinite sine waves have a single frequency. The beginning and end of an ultrasound pulse introduce a range of frequencies; the shorter the pulse, the wider its frequency spectrum. A "high Q" transducer will respond to a short voltage pulse with a relatively long-lasting vibration, emitting ultrasound with a narrow bandwidth (nearly "pure" sound). A "low Q" transducer, on the other hand, will vibrate for only a short time period, emitting a short pulse of ultrasound consisting of a broad range of frequencies. Adding a backing block to an ultrasound transducer reduces the Q factor by shortening the ringdown time and consequently the pulse duration, which increases the bandwidth of the ultrasound pulse. "Low Q" transducers are preferable in ultrasound imaging systems where a small spatial pulse length is needed for high axial resolution. Doppler ultrasound applications require transducers with higher Q factor to produce narrow bandwidth ultrasound which is needed for detection of the frequency changes caused by blood flow.

SPATIAL PULSE LENGTH

The length of the ultrasound pulse in pulsed ultrasound applications. The spatial pulse length is equal to the number of waves (cycles) in the pulse multiplied by their wavelength. The pulse length is determined by the Q factor of the transducer crystal and by the characteristics of the backing block of the transducer. The spatial pulse length determines the axial resolution of the pulsed ultrasound system.

AXIAL RESOLUTION

The spatial resolution of ultrasound in the ultrasound beam direction, also known as the depth, linear, longitudinal and range resolution. The axial resolution is the minimum distance in the beam direction between two reflectors which can be identified as separate echoes. The axial resolution is slightly more than half the spatial pulse length, which is the number of waves in the transmitted ultrasound pulse (determined by the Q factor) multiplied by their wavelength (determined by the transducer frequency).

ARTEFACT IN ULTRASOUND

display of incorrect anatomy or velocity in ultrasound applications. In B mode imaging, artefacts may appear whenever there is a violation of the following assumptions:

1.	The ultrasound beam is narrow with uniform width.
2.	The speed of sound is 1540 m/s in soft tissues.
3.	The attenuation of ultrasound is uniform.
4.	The ultrasound travels in a straight line directly to the reflecting object and back to the transducer.
5.	Echoes from all depths are allowed to reach the transducer before the next ultrasound pulse is emitted.

Assumption 1) may be violated by a wide beam, which causes image smearing of echogenic objects that are smaller than the beam diameter (beam width artefact), or by side lobes or grating lobes (side lobe artefact). Assumption 2) that the speed of sound is constant at 1 540 m/s, is true for most soft tissues, but it is lower in fat (1 450 m/s) and especially in silicone implants (600 m/s). This causes errors in range and distance, and may cause the so-called speed artefact. Variations in attenuation (assumption 3) may cause artificially increased image brightness (enhancement

artefact) or decreased image brightness (shadowing artefact). Several artefacts are caused by violation of assumption 4, such as the mirror image artefact or multipath reflection artefact, the reverberation artefact (also named ring-down artefact or comet tail artefact), and split image artefact. Assumption 5 may be violated by a too high pulse repetition frequency PRF, giving rise to the ambiguity artefact.

In Doppler ultrasound applications, artefacts appear whenever the Doppler frequency shift exceeds the Nyquist limit. This causes aliasing, which may be seen as frequency fold over or frequency wrap around in spectral Doppler, or as a mosaic effect in colour Doppler sonography. Use of gas microbubble contrast media may cause bubble noise and blooming artefact.

SHADOWING ARTEFACT

In ultrasound imaging, a hypoechoic (dark) area distal to an object. The low signal is caused by attenuation (absorption, reflection or refraction) of the ultrasound beam. Shadowing artefacts are typically seen as dark streaking behind highly attenuating objects such as bones and calculi (in e.g. gall bladder or kidney). Dark streaks are also seen distal to the lateral borders of fluid-containing structures (e.g. gall bladder, cysts) due to reflection and refraction of the ultrasound beam from the curved surface.

AMBIGUITY ARTEFACT

Ultrasound image artefact occurring when the pulse repetition frequency PRF is too high to allow the deepest echoes to return to the transducer before the next ultrasound pulse is transmitted. The deepest echoes arrive at the transducer shortly after the next pulse transmission and are consequently mismapped to shallow positions in the image.

BLOOMING ARTEFACT

Smearing of colour signals outside a vessel in colour Doppler sonography, caused by gas microbubble contrast medium. The phenomenon may be due to multiple reflections of the ultrasound back and forth between the bubbles, similar to the reverberation artefact of B mode imaging, and perhaps also to high amplitude echoes caused by collapse of the microbubbles in the ultrasound beam.

Key Points

Absorption is the transfer of energy from the ultrasound beam to the tissue. It is proportional to frequency.

Apodization is a method for reducing side lobes in some arrays. It gradually decreases the vibration of the transducer surface with distance from its center. It is usually accomplished by using more power to excite the innermost elements.

Axial resolution is the minimum separation between two interfaces located in a direction parallel to the beam so that they can be imaged as two different interfaces.

Decibel is a way to express the ratio of two sound intensities: $dB = 10\log_{10}I1/I2$ being I1 the reference. For instance: +3 dB = I multiplied by 2 and -3 db = I divided by 2

Diffraction is the change in the directions and intensities of a group of waves after passing by an obstacle or through an aperture.

Duty factor is the lapse of time the transducer is actively transmitting sound.

Echo ranging is the relationship between transit time and reflector depth expressed as $t = 2d/c$.

Grating lobes as side lobes are secondary ultrasound beams projecting off-axis at predictable angles to the main beam. Side lobes are too small to produce important artifacts.

Half Value Layer (HVL) is the distance the sound beam penetrates into a tissue when its intensity has been reduced to one half of its initial value.

Huygens' principle states that an expanding sphere of waves behaves as if each point on the wave front were a new source of radiation of the same frequency and phase.

Impedance is the product of the density of a material and the speed of sound in that material.

Pulse average intensity I(PA) is the average intensity during the pulse.

Lateral resolution is the minimum separation of two interfaces aligned along a direction perpendicular to the ultrasound beam. It depends on the beam width.

Partial Volume Artifact (slice thickness or volume averaging artifact), that occurs when the slice thickness is wider than the scanned structure.

Q-value means the degree that a transducer is finely tuned to specific narrow frequency range. For instance: Low Q means wide bandwitdh and High Q means narrow bandwidth.

Range resolution is the ability to determine the depth of reflectors.

Rayleigh scatterers are objects whose dimensions are much less than the ultrasound wavelength. Scattering increases with frequency raised to the 4th power and provides much of the diagnostic information from ultrasound.

Refraction is the bending of a wave beam when it crosses at an oblique angle the interface of two materials, through which the waves propagate at different velocities

Snell's law governs the direction of the transmitted beam when refraction occurs:

sin qt = (c2/c1) x sin qi (qt and qi are transmit and incident angles respectively)

Spatial Average Intensity (SA) is the acoustic power within the beam, divided by the beam area.

Spatial Peak Intensity (SP) is the point in the sound field with maximum intensity.

Side lobes are energy in the sound beam falling outside the main beam.

Spatial resolution means how closely two reflectors -or scattering regions, can be to one another while they can be identified as different reflectors.

Subdicing is a technique used to overcome grating lobes: each major transducer element is divided into smaller parts, each one being a half wave length.

Temporal (instantaneous) Peak Intensity I(TP) or I(IP) is the maximum intensity during the pulse.

Time Average Intensity I(TA): average intensity calculated over the time between pulses:

$$ITA = I(PA) \times Duty\ factor.$$

Wavelength is l=c/f (c = propagation speed; f = frequency)

Ultrasound Physics

Ultrasound, unlike light and x-rays, needs a medium for travel. For our purposes, this propagating medium is tissue or fluid. Ultrasound cannot travel though air, even the smallest amount. Air is therefore an acoustic barrier while the presence of fluid is quite helpful for sonograms. This is exactly the opposite of radiology, where air is "our friend", yielding contrast, while fluid is "our enemy" obscuring organs from view. Diagnostic ultrasound utilizes sound waves at a very high frequency, in the range of 2-10 megahertz (MHz). This is in contrast to audible sound which is in the 20-20,000 Hz range.

Diagnostic ultrasound utilizes the "pulse echo" principle to create a visible image of tissue and tissue interfaces within the body. An electrical impulse is applied to a piezoelectric (pressure electric) crystal or crystals within the transducer (probe). These crystals convert electrical energy into mechanical energy (ultrasound). The ultrasound travels within the soft tissues of the body at an average of 1540 m/sec. As the sound reaches each organ or tissue, a portion of the sound is reflected (echoes) back to the transducer, which now converts the mechanical energy (returning ultrasound) into electrical energy. This electrical information is then processed by the computer within the ultrasound machine, forming an image on the display screen. The image on the screen is created by a multitude of "dots", each dot located at the appropriate depth of the reflected echo, determined by how long it took for that particular echo to return to the transducer. The brightness or whiteness of each dot is determined by the strength of the returning echo. No returning echoes from a particular location are depicted as black dots (anechoic). The pulses of sound emitted by the transducer occur only 0.1% of the time, allowing the transducer to listen for returning echoes 99.9% of the time. This is an important concept, as the biological effects of ultrasound (heat deposition in tissue) have proven to be negligible since very little time is spent transmitting the ultrasound beam. This is in contrast to therapeutic ultrasound, which utilizes continuous transmission of ultrasound.

As ultrasound travels through tissue, it grows weaker (diminished volume), known as attenuation. Attenuation occurs by three processes. Absorption occurs when the energy is captured by the tissue and converted to heat. Scattering occurs when the ultrasound beam encounters irregular interfaces, sending it in all directions (thus only a small percentage of it returns to the transducer to contribute to image formation). Reflection of sound is the third process in attenuation of the ultrasound beam, occurring at interfaces between tissues of different acoustic properties. The net effect is attenuation of approximately 0.5 dB/cm/MHZ. Higher frequency ultrasound is attenuated more rapidly over distance traveled than lower frequencies. Therefore, lower frequency transducers (e.g., 2.5 MHz) are used to image deeper structures. Higher frequency transducers (e.g., 7.5 MHz) offer much better resolution at the expense of less depth penetration.

TERMINOLOGY

Ultrasound terminology describes organs or structures as to how echogenic they are relative to other tissues in the same patient. The following are those most commonly used:

Hypoechoic-less intense echo production (object appears darker gray)

Hyperechoic-more intense or more highly reflective (object appears lighter gray to white)

Anechoic-absence of echoes (objects appear black)

Isoechoic-of the dame echogenicity

Mixed echogenicity-having a complex echo pattern of two or more echogenicities

The relative echogenicities of normal abdominal organs from least echogenic (darkest) to most echogenic (brightest, whitest) are:

renal medulla<renal cortex<liver<spleen<prostate gland

Spatial resolution is the ability to identify two closely spaced objects. The smaller the distance that can be separated, the better the resolution. Axial resolution is the ability to resolve closely spaced objects along the axis of the ultrasound beam. Lateral resolution is the ability to resolve closely spaced objects perpendicular to the ultrasound beam's axis (side-by-side). Axial resolution is greater than lateral resolution.

ARTIFACTS

Distant Enhancement - an artifact that occurs deep to fluid-filled structures (e.g., gallbladder), resulting in brighter echoes because the ultrasound is not attenuated by the fluid.

Acoustic Shadowing - failure of the ultrasound beam to pass through an object because of reflection and/or absorption of the ultrasound. The result is an anechoic (black) zone beyond the surface of the reflector. This occurs with mineral or gas (e.g., bone, cystic calculus, lung.)

Reverberation - an artifact that is the result of sound bouncing back and forth between two interfaces, resulting in repeated time delays and the display of parallel lines at regular intervals deep to the actual returning echo. This is the common artifact seen when imaging aerated lung or gas within a loop of intestine or stomach. Ring-down artifacts, occurring at the skin-transducer surface and comet-tail artifacts, which occur with metal or air interfaces are other common examples of reverberation artifact.

Refraction - a bending or change in direction of the ultrasound beam as it encounters a rounded structure resulting in an area of echo drop-out, mimicking an acoustic shadow. This commonly occurs along the edge of the kidney, or from within the kidney at the corticomedullary junction.

Mirror-image - artifactual image appearing on the opposite side of a strong, curved reflector, the result of multiple internal reverberations between the object and the reflector, creating a time delay in the return of these internal echoes to the transducer. Thus, an erroneously placed structure in addition to the "real" structure is displayed on the video screen. The common mirror-image artifact is the liver and gallbladder, seen on the "other side" of the diaphragm. This could be mistaken for a diaphragmatic hernia.

Four types of Doppler Ultrasound

CONTINUOUS WAVE (CW)

This mode requires a transducer with separate elements for transmitting and receiving. Because of the continuous wave of ultrasound, a single transducer element cannot alternate between transmitting and receiving. CW ultrasound does not have the ability to discriminate depth of velocities. It samples velocities all along its path. Its primary use is to accurately measure high blood flows, such as across a stenotic valve, which pulse wave and color Doppler are unable to do.

PULSE WAVE (PW)

The principal advantage of a PW Doppler is that blood flow velocity can be determined at a specific site. Limitations are that it is cannot measure high velocities (due to the Nyquist limit, called aliasing).

CW and PW Doppler are displayed on a x-y axis, known as spectral Doppler. Each vertical line in the display represents a specific instant in time. The length represents the range of velocities present. The top of the line indicates the maximum velocity. Sound can be used to listen to blood flow as well.

COLOR

Color Doppler is form of PW Doppler and thus subject to the same limitations of high velocity. The display color is determined by the direction and relative flow velocity. Typically, the color display is superimposed on a conventional B-mode. In a typical color Doppler display, red indicates flow toward the transducer and blue indicates flow in the opposite direction. Other colors represent turbulence or aliasing artifact.

ENERGY OR POWER DOPPLER

This is the newest form of Doppler. It is capable of detecting the smallest of blood flow. However, there is no display of velocity or direction. It allows the visualization of smaller vessels. It contains only one color scale and produces a homogeneous color appearance overlying a B-mode image. Power Doppler is only available on sophisticated and very expensive equipment.

PIEZOELECTRIC EFFECT

The phenomenon that certain crystals change their physical dimensions when subjected to an electric field, and vice versa; when deformed by external pressure, an electric field is created across the crystal (from the Greek word piezein = pressure). Piezoelectric crystals are used in ultrasound transducers to transmit and receive ultrasound.

EFFECT OF APPLIED ELECTRIC FIELD

The piezoelectric crystal in ultrasound transducers has electrodes attached to its front and back for the application and detection of electrical charges. The crystal consists of numerous dipoles, and in the normal state, the individual dipoles have an oblique orientation with no net surface charge. An electric field applied across the crystal will realign the dipoles due to repulsive or attractive electric forces resulting in compression or expansion of the crystal, depending on the direction of the electric field. (For transmission of a short ultrasound pulse, a voltage spike of very short duration is applied, causing the crystal to initially contract and then vibrate for a short time with its resonant frequency.)

EFFECT OF EXTERNAL PRESSURE

When echoes are received, the longitudinal ultrasound waves will compress and expand the crystal. This deformation realigns the dipoles, creating net charges on the crystal surface. In practice, the compression and expansion only amount to a few microns.

Sensitivity in Ultrasound

IMPORTANCE OF HIGH SENSITIVITY

Higher sensitivity (larger d_1 or g_1 constant) represents a larger response and improved signal-to-noise ratio for a given stimulus. Selecting the proper piezoelectric material for a given application often involves a trade-off between sensitivity and other properties such as Curie point or Dielectric constant. For example, materials with the highest charge constant (d_1) have lower Curie points than materials with lower charge constants.

NEED OF HIGH SENSITIVITY IN MEDICAL ULTRASOUND

The piezoelectric material both projects and senses the acoustic wave. High sensitivity is necessary to maximize the signal-to-noise ratio for the returned acoustic wave.

Piezoelectricity

In 1880, Jacques and Pierre Curie discovered an unusual characteristic of certain crystalline minerals: when subjected to a mechanical force, the crystals became electrically polarized. Tension and compression generated voltages of opposite polarity, and in proportion to the applied force. Subsequently, the converse of this relationship was confirmed: if one of these voltage-generating crystals was exposed to an electric field it lengthened or shortened according to the polarity of the field, and in proportion to the strength of the field. These behaviors were labeled the piezoelectric effect and the inverse piezoelectric effect, respectively, from the Greek word piezein, meaning to press or squeeze.

Although the magnitudes of piezoelectric voltages, movements, or forces are small, and often require amplification (a typical disc of piezoelectric ceramic will increase or decrease in thickness by only a small fraction of a millimeter, for example) piezoelectric materials have been adapted to an impressive range of applications. The piezoelectric effect is used in sensing applications, such as in force or displacement sensors. The inverse piezoelectric effect is used in actuation applications, such as in motors and devices that precisely control positioning, and in generating sonic and ultrasonic signals.

In the 20th century metal oxide-based piezoelectric ceramics and other man-made materials enabled designers to employ the piezoelectric effect and the inverse piezoelectric effect in many new applications. These materials generally are physically strong and chemically inert, and they are relatively inexpensive to manufacture. The composition, shape, and dimensions of a piezoelectric ceramic element can be tailored to meet the requirements of a specific purpose. Ceramics manufactured from formulations of lead zirconate / lead titanate exhibit greater sensitivity and higher operating temperatures, relative to ceramics of other compositions, and "PZT" materials currently are the most widely used piezoelectric ceramics.

MAKING OF PIEZOELECTRIC CERAMICS

A traditional piezoelectric ceramic is a mass of perovskite crystals, each consisting of a small, tetravalent metal ion, usually titanium or zirconium, in a lattice of larger, divalent metal ions, usually lead or barium, and O^{2-} ions. Under conditions that confer tetragonal or rhombohedral symmetry on the crystals, each crystal has a dipole moment.

To prepare a piezoelectric ceramic, fine powders of the component metal oxides are mixed in specific proportions, then heated to form a uniform powder. The powder is mixed with an organic binder and is formed into structural elements having the desired shape (discs, rods, plates, etc.). The elements are fired according to a specific time and temperature program, during which the powder particles sinter and the material attains a dense crystalline structure. The elements are cooled, then shaped or trimmed to specifications, and electrodes are applied to the appropriate surfaces.

Above a critical temperature, the *Curie point*, each perovskite crystal in the fired ceramic element exhibits a simple cubic symmetry with no dipole moment. At temperatures below the Curie point, however, each crystal has tetragonal or rhombohedral symmetry and a dipole moment. Adjoining dipoles form regions of local alignment called *domains*. The alignment gives a net dipole moment to the domain, and thus a net polarization. The direction of polarization among neighboring domains is random, however, so the ceramic element has no overall polarization.

The domains in a ceramic element are aligned by exposing the element to a strong, direct current electric field, usually at a temperature slightly below the Curie point. Through this polarizing *(poling)* treatment, domains most nearly aligned with the electric field expand at the expense of domains that are not aligned with the field, and the element lengthens in the direction of the field. When the electric field is removed most of the dipoles are locked into a configuration of near alignment. The element now has a permanent polarization, the remnant polarization, and is permanently elongated.

FUNCTION OF PIEZOELECTRIC CERAMICS

Mechanical compression or tension on a poled piezoelectric ceramic element changes the dipole moment, creating a voltage. Compression along the direction of polarization, or tension perpendicular to the direction of polarization, generates voltage of the same polarity as the poling voltage. Tension along the direction of polarization, or compression perpendicular to the direction of polarization, generates a voltage with polarity opposite that of the poling voltage. These actions are generator actions -- the ceramic element converts the mechanical energy of compression or tension into electrical energy. This behavior is used in fuel-igniting devices, solid state batteries, force-sensing devices, and other products. Values for compressive stress and the voltage (or field strength) generated by applying stress to a piezoelectric ceramic element are linearly proportional up to a material-specific stress. The same is true for applied voltage and generated strain.

If a voltage of the same polarity as the poling voltage is applied to a ceramic element, in the direction of the poling voltage, the element will lengthen and its diameter will become smaller. If a voltage of polarity opposite that of the poling voltage is applied, the element will become shorter and broader. If an alternating voltage is applied, the element will lengthen and shorten cyclically, at the frequency of the applied voltage. This is motor action -- electrical energy is converted into mechanical energy. The principle is adapted to piezoelectric motors, sound or ultrasound generating devices, and many other products.

Properties of Acoustic Plane Wave

WAVELENGTH, FREQUENCY AND VELOCITY

Among the properties of waves propagating in isotropic solid materials are wavelength, frequency, and velocity. The wavelength is directly proportional to the velocity of the wave and inversely proportional to the frequency of the wave. This relationship is shown by the following equation.

$$\text{Wavelength}(\lambda) = \frac{\text{Velocity}(v)}{\text{Frequency}(f)}$$

REFRACTION AND SNELL'S LAW

When an ultrasound wave passes through an interface between two materials at an oblique angle, and the materials have different indices of refraction, it produces both reflected and refracted waves. This also occurs with light and this makes objects you see across an interface appear to be shifted relative to where they really are. For example, if you look straight down at an object at the bottom of a glass of water, it looks closer than it really is. A good way to visualize how light and sound refract is to shine a flashlight into a bowl of slightly cloudy water noting the refraction angle with respect to the incidence angle.

Refraction takes place at an interface due to the different velocities of the acoustic waves within the two materials. The velocity of sound in each material is determined by the material properties (elastic modules and density) for that material. In the animation below, a series of plane waves are shown traveling in one material and entering a second material that has a higher acoustic velocity. Therefore, when the wave encounters the interface between these two materials, the portion of the wave in the second material is moving faster than the portion of the wave in the first material. It can be seen that this causes the wave to bend.

Snell's Law describes the relationship between the angles and the velocities of the waves. Snell's law equates the ratio of material velocities **v1** and **v2** to the ratio of the **sine's** of incident (θ_1) and refraction (θ_2) angles, as shown in the following equation.

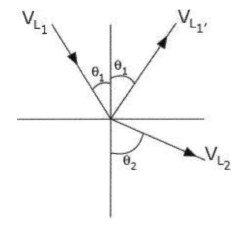

$$\frac{sin\theta_1}{V_{L_1}} = \frac{sin\theta_2}{V_{L_2}}$$

Where:
V_{L1} is the longitudinal wave velocity in material 1.
V_{L2} is the longitudinal wave velocity in material 2.

Note that in the diagram, there is a reflected longitudinal wave (V_{L_1}) shown. This wave is reflected at the same angle as the incident wave because the two waves are traveling in the same material and, therefore, have the same velocities. This reflected wave is unimportant in our explanation of Snell's Law, but it should be remembered that some of the wave energy is reflected at the interface.

Piezoelectric Transducers

The conversion of electrical pulses to mechanical vibrations and the conversion of returned mechanical vibrations back into electrical energy is the basis for ultrasonic testing. The active element is the heart of the transducer as it converts the electrical energy to acoustic energy, and vice versa. The active element is basically a piece polarized material (i.e. some parts of the molecule are positively charged, while other parts of the molecule are negatively charged) with electrodes attached to two of its opposite faces. When an electric field is applied across the material, the polarized molecules will align themselves with the electric field, resulting in induced dipoles within the molecular or crystal structure of the material. This alignment of molecules will cause the material to change dimensions. This phenomenon is known as electrostriction. In addition, a permanently-polarized material such as quartz (SiO_2) or barium titanate ($BaTiO_3$) will produce an electric field when the material changes dimensions as a result of an imposed mechanical force. This phenomenon is known as the piezoelectric effect.

The thickness of the active element is determined by the desired frequency of the transducer. A thin wafer element vibrates with a wavelength that is twice its thickness. Therefore, piezoelectric crystals are cut to a thickness that is 1/2 the desired radiated wavelength. The higher the frequency of the transducer, the thinner the active element. The primary reason that high frequency contact transducers are not produced in because the element is very thin and too fragile.

72

Characteristics of Piezoelectric Transducers

The transducer is a very important part of the ultrasonic instrumentation system. As discussed on the previous page, the transducer incorporates a piezoelectric element, which converts electrical signals into mechanical vibrations (transmit mode) and mechanical vibrations into electrical signals (receive mode). Many factors, including material, mechanical and electrical construction, and the external mechanical and electrical load conditions, influence the behavior a transducer. Mechanical construction includes parameters such as radiation surface area, mechanical damping, housing, connector type and other variables of physical construction. As of this writing, transducer manufactures are hard pressed when constructing two transducers that have identical performance characteristics.

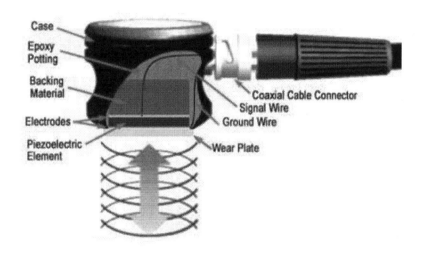

A cut away of a typical contact transducer is shown above. It was previously learned that the piezoelectric element is cut to 1/2 the desired wavelength. To get as much energy out of the transducer as possible, an impedance matching is placed between the active element and the face of the transducer. Optimal impedance matching is achieved by sizing the matching layer so that its thickness is 1/4 wavelength. This keeps waves that were reflected within the matching layer in phase when they exit the layer as illustrated in the image to the right. For contact transducers, the matching layer is made from a material that has an acoustical impedance between the active element and steel. Immersion transducers have a matching layer with an acoustical impedance between the active element and water. Contact transducers also often incorporate a wear plate to protect the matching layer and active element from scratch.

The backing material supporting the crystal has a great influence on damping characteristics of a transducer. Using a backing material with an impedance similar to that of the active element will produce the most effective damping. Such a transducer will have a narrow bandwidth resulting in higher sensitivity. As the mismatch in impedance between the active element and the backing material increases, material penetration increased but transducer sensitivity is reduced.

Transducer Efficiency, Bandwidth and Frequency

Some transducers are specially fabricated to be more efficient transmitters and others to be more efficient receivers. A transducer that performs well in one application will not always produce the desired results in a different application. For example, sensitivity to small defects is proportional to the product of the efficiency of the transducer as a transmitter and a receiver. Resolution, the ability to locate defects near surface or in close proximity in the material, requires a highly damped transducer.

It is also important to understand the concept of bandwidth, or range of frequencies, associated with a transducer. The frequency noted on a transducer is the central or center frequency and depends primarily on the backing material. Highly damped transducers will respond to frequencies above and below the central frequency. The broad frequency range provides a transducer with high resolving power. Less damped transducers will exhibit a narrower frequency range, poorer resolving power, but greater penetration.

Transducers are constructed to withstand some abuse, but they should be handled carefully. Misuse such as dropping can cause cracking of the wear plate, element, or the backing material. Damage to a transducer is often noted on the a-scan presentation as an enlargement of the initial pulse.

Transducer Beam Spread

Round transducers are often referred to as piston source transducers because the sound field resembles a cylindrical mass in front of the transducer. However, the energy in the beam does not remain in a cylinder, but instead spread out as it propagates through the material. The phenomenon is usually referred to as beam spread but is sometimes also called beam divergence or ultrasonic diffraction. Although beam spread must be considered when performing an ultrasonic inspection, it is important to note that in the far field, or Fraunhofer zone, the maximum sound pressure is always found along the acoustic axis (centerline) of the transducer. Therefore, the strongest reflection is likely to come from the area directly in front of the transducer.

Beam spread occurs because the vibrating particle of the material (through which the wave is traveling) do not always transfer all of their energy in the direction of wave propagation. Recall that waves propagate through that transfer of energy from one particle to another in the medium. If the particles are not directly aligned in the direction of wave propagation, some of the energy will get transferred off at an angle. (Picture what happens when one ball hits another second ball slightly off center). In the near field constructive and destructive wave interference fill the sound field with fluctuation. At the start of the far field, however, the beam strength is always greatest at the center of the beam and diminishes as it spreads outward.

Beam spread is greater when using a low frequency transducer than when using a high frequency transducer. As the diameter of the transducer increases the beam spread will be reduced.

Transducer Testing

As part of the documentation process, an extensive database containing records of the waveform and spectrum of each transducer is maintained and can be accessed for comparative or statistical studies of transducer characteristics.

Manufactures often provide time and frequency domain plots for each transducer. The signals below were generated by a spiked pulser. The waveform image on the left shows the test response signal in the time domain (amplitude versus time). The spectrum image on the right shows the same signal in the frequency domain (amplitude versus frequency). The signal path is usually a reflection from the back wall (fused silica) with the reflection in the far field of the transducer.

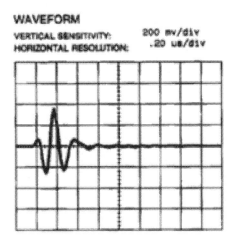

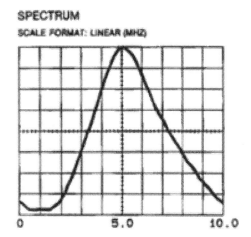

Other tests may include the following:

- **Electrical Impedance Plots** provide important information about the design and construction of a transducer and can allow users to obtain electrically similar transducers from multiple sources.
- **Beam Alignment Measurements** provide data on the degree of alignment between the sound beam axis and the transducer housing. This information is particularly useful in applications that require a high degree of certainty regarding beam positioning with respect to a mechanical reference surface.
- **Beam Profiles** provide valuable information about transducer sound field characteristics. Transverse beam profiles are created by scanning the transducer across a target (usually either a steel ball or rod) at a given distance from the transducer face and are used to determine focal spot size and beam symmetry. Axial beam profiles are created by recording the pulse-echo amplitude of the sound field as a function of distance from the transducer face and provide data on depth of field and focal length.

AXIAL RESOLUTION

The spatial resolution of ultrasound in the ultrasound beam direction, also known as the depth, linear, longitudinal and range resolution. The axial resolution is the minimum distance in the beam direction between two reflectors which can be identified as separate echoes. The axial resolution is slightly more than half the spatial pulse length, which is the number of waves in the transmitted ultrasound pulse (determined by the Q factor) multiplied by their wavelength (determined by the transducer frequency).

DIGITAL SCAN CONVERTER

A component of all modern ultrasound imaging instruments that digitizes the scanned information and converts the ultrasound echoes into a two-dimensional B mode image composed of pixels. The digital scan converter is composed of an analogue to digital converter ADC, a computer and computer memory, and a digital to analogue converter DAC. In most ultrasound instruments, the ADC digitizes the echo amplitudes into 6 or 7 bits, i.e. 26 (64) or 27 (128) grey levels. The digital information is stored in the computer memory as a digital matrix, usually composed of $512 \cdot 512$ pixels. Each digitized echo is positioned in the matrix according to transducer or transducer element position (determining the horizontal pixel position), and to the time lapse from pulse transmission to echo detection (determining the vertical or depth position in the matrix). The DAC converts this true digital image into an analogue image on a TV monitor, by assigning each pixel in the analogue image a brightness determined by the digital number of the pixel in the digital image matrix.

ANALOGUE-TO-DIGITAL CONVERTER (ADC)

Electronic device which converts the analogue audiofrequency signals from, for example, an MR or ultrasound receiver into digital form so that it can be stored and processed by the computer. Important parameters for determining the performance of an ADC include the sampling speed and word length.

The Doppler Equation

This Doppler effect in tissues maybe expressed as an equation as shown in this figure. Simply stated, the Doppler shift (Fd) of ultrasound will depend on both the transmitted frequency (fo) and the velocity (V) of the moving blood. This returned frequency is also called the "frequency shift" or "Doppler shift" and is highly dependent upon the angle (?) between the beam of ultrasound transmitted from the transducer and the moving red blood cells. The velocity of sound in blood is constant (c) and is an important part of the Doppler equation.

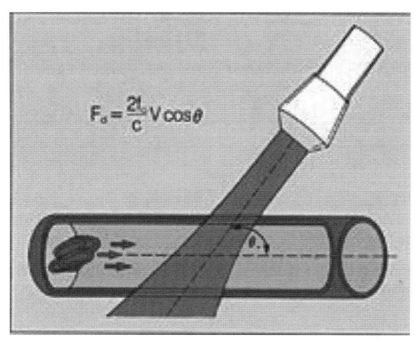

$$F_d = \frac{2f_o}{c} V \cos\theta$$

Doppler Key Points

Aliasing is an artifact that lowers the frequency components when the PRF is less than 2 times the highest frequency of a Doppler signal

Beat frequency, for CW Doppler, is the Doppler shift

Ensemble length -packet size, shots per line- is the number of pulses per scan line. In color Doppler, each line of sight most be pulsed several times

FFT. Fast Fourier Transform analyzer is a common device that performs spectral analysis in ultrasound instruments. In this case, it displays different quadrature Doppler frequencies, or reflector velocities when a sample volume cursor is used (Doppler frequency is proportional to reflector velocity) along time

High pass filter is the wall filter

Nyquist Frequency is the maximum frequency that can be sampled without aliasing. NF = PRF/2 (PRF stands for Pulse Repetition Frequency)

Quadrature detection is a signal processing method for directional Doppler in which the signal reference frequency for two channels differ in phase by 1/4 period. The output Doppler signal phase for both channels also depends on the Doppler shift, whether positive or negative

Spectral analysis is the quantitative analysis to display the distribution of frequencies

Variance is the variation of Doppler frequencies within each pixel during a pulse packet, effective to detect turbulence with color Doppler

The Doppler Principle

DIRECTION AND VELOCITY OF FLOW

The fact that makes frequency of the Doppler effect more than just an interesting curiosity is that it actually provides a method that is used to measure the direction and speed of moving red blood cells. Clinically we are most interested in measuring velocity since, as mentioned above, it is altered in disease states.

A Doppler system then compares the transmitted waveform with the received waveform for a change in frequency. These are called "phase shifts" and they are automatically determined within the Doppler instrument. If there is a higher returning frequency (+AP) then the flow is called a "positive Doppler shift" and represented as moving toward the transducer. If there is a lower returning frequency (-AP) then the flow is called a "negative Doppler shift" and represented as moving away from the transducer. All components of the Doppler equation, except velocity, are readily measured by the Doppler instrument.

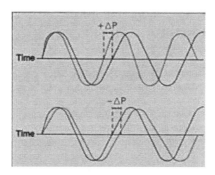

The Doppler equation may be rearranged to solve for velocity of blood movement. The angle may be measured or may be assumed to be parallel depending upon orientation of the beam by the system operator.

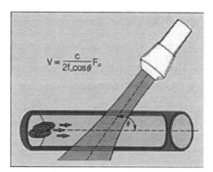

The Doppler device can be regarded as a complex speedometer designed to detect red cell motion (i.e., blood flow) and measure its velocity. What is important to recognize is that:

> FREQUENCY SHIFT >>> DOPPLER EQUATION >>> VELOCITY DATA

81

THE DOPPLER DISPLAY

All Doppler systems have audio outputs and listening to this is very helpful during a Doppler examination. The changing velocities (frequencies) are converted into audible sounds and, after some processing, are emitted from speakers placed within the machine.

High pitched sounds result from large Doppler shifts and indicate the presence of high velocities, while low pitched sounds result from lesser Doppler shifts. Flow direction information (relative to the transducer) is provided by a stereophonic audio output in which flow toward the transducer comes out of one speaker and flow away from the transducer.

The audio output also allows the operator to easily differentiate laminar from turbulent flow. Laminar flow produces a smooth, pleasant tone because of the uniform velocities. Turbulent flow, because of the presence of many different velocities, results in a commonly high-pitched and whistling or harsh and raspy sound.

The audio output remains an indispensable guide to the machine operator for achieving proper orientation of the ultrasound beam, even when Doppler echocardiography is being used in conjunction with an ultrasound imaging technique. The trained ear can readily appreciate minor changes in spectral composition more readily than the eye, given the same information displayed graphically. The major limitation of audio Doppler outputs is the requirements for subjective interpretation and the lack of a permanent objective record. The audio output from a Doppler machine is not the same as that received by a stethoscope or a phonocardiogram. The sounds detected with a stethoscope are transmitted vibrations or pressure waves from the heart and great vessels that are believed to be the result of rapid accelerations and decelerations of blood. The Doppler audio output, in contrast, is an audible display of the Doppler frequency shift spectrum produced by red cells moving in the path of the ultrasound beam. It is a sound produced by the Doppler machine that does not occur in nature and, therefore, it does not originate in the heart.

All newer generations of Doppler echocardiography equipment contain sophisticated sound frequency or velocity spectrum analyzers for hard copy recording. Most commercially available Doppler systems display a spectrum of the various velocities present at any time and are, therefore, called "spectral velocity recordings.

Flow velocity toward the transducer is displayed as a positive, or upward, shift in velocities while flow velocity away from the transducer is displayed as a negative, or downward shift in velocities. Time is on the horizontal axis.

The internal working of such systems is complex but the results are rather simple. When flow is laminar and all the red cells are accelerating and decelerating at approximately the same velocities, a neat envelope of these similar velocities is recorded over time. When flow is turbulent, however, there are many different velocities detected at any one time (a wide spectrum of velocities). Such turbulence, produced by an obstruction to flow, results in the spectral broadening (display of velocities that are low, mid and high) and an increase in peak velocity as seen in disease states.

This display of the spectrum of the various velocities encountered by the Doppler beam is accomplished by very sophisticated microcomputers that are able to decode the returning complex Doppler signal and process it into its various velocity components. There are two basic methods for accomplishing this. The most popular is Fast Fourier Transform (FFT) and the other is called Chirp-Z Transform. These are simply ways for deciphering, analyzing and presenting vast amounts of returning data

THE EFFECT OF ANGLE

The Doppler equation also tells us that the angle the Doppler beam is relative to the lines of flow being evaluated is very important.

When the ultrasound beam is directed parallel to blood flow, angle θ (cosine 0° = 1) and measured velocity on the recording will be true velocity. In contrast, with the ultrasound beam directed perpendicular to flow, angle θ = 90 degrees (cosine 90° = 0) and measured velocity will be zero. Therefore, the smaller the angle, the closer angle cosine θ is to 1.0 and the more reliable is the recorded Doppler velocity. A wider angle will result in a greater reduction in measured velocity compared to true velocity.

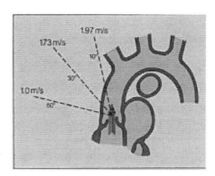

Thus, the more parallel to flow the Doppler ultrasound beam is directed the more faithfully the measured velocity will reflect true velocity. For practical purposes, angles of greater than 25° between the ultrasound beam and the blood flow being studied will generally yield clinically unacceptable qualitative estimates of velocity.

Color Flow Imaging in Clinical Practice

THE MEANING OF COLOR

The colors displayed on the flow map image contain useful information. By convention, Doppler color flow systems assign a given color to the direction of flow; red is flow toward, and blue is flow away from the transducer. Three typical color bars from a color flow imaging device are shown in the figure and give an initial frame of reference to the meaning of colors. Such color reference bars always appear on the screen of Doppler flow imaging devices. The center of the standard color bar on the left is black (white center reference mark) and represents zero flow.

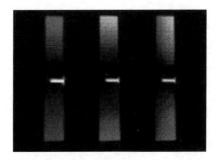

In addition to simple direction, velocity information is also displayed. Progressively increasing velocities are encoded in varying hues of either red or blue. The more dull the hue, the slower the velocity. The brighter the hue, the faster the relative velocity.

COLOR FLOW IMAGING IN CLINICAL PRACTICE
THE ANGIOGRAPHIC CONCEPT

One way of conceptualizing Doppler color flow methods is to recognize its similarity to angiography. It provides a noninvasive "angiogram" of blood flow, where the contrast medium is the moving red blood cells and the detector of this contrast is ultrasound. The complex Doppler ultrasound processing circuitry allows for the detection of movement of these red cells in various directions - forward and backward through the heart. Doppler color flow information, however, is obtained and displayed in a cross-sectional image, making the spatial details of flow and anatomy readily recognizable. In effect, Doppler color flow looks inside the cineangiographic silhouette.

CREATION OF THE COLOR IMAGE
THE IMPORTANCE OF TIME

Time is the key factor to keep in mind. A conventional two-dimensional ultrasound imaging system is already working as hard as it can. Pulses must be transmitted along a given line, reflected from the heart valves and walls, then received. The process is repeated, line by line, through the entire sector arc that comprises several hundred lines. This completes one frame of information, usually in one-thirtieth of a second. In order to have the image appear as though it is continuously moving, the entire image must be updated 30 times in a second (30 frames/second). This results in relatively long waiting periods for the transmit-receive sequence to be completed. It also means that considerable amounts of information need to be quickly processed and presented in the image.

Creation of the Color Image

Expressed in its most simplistic terms, color flow systems add a separate processor that creates the color flow image based on the returning data and then integrates it with the two-dimensional anatomic image. Both the anatomic and the color flow data are then displayed in the final image.

The returning ultrasound data from any conventional scanner also contains frequency shift information that results from the encounter of the transmitted pulse with moving structures and blood. Until the advent of color flow imaging, this frequency shift data was simply ignored.

The key to color flow mapping is that the returning data may also be processed for the frequency shifts (or red blood cell velocities). Thus, color flow imaging systems take advantage of data that are available in every ultrasound image of the heart.

While this is a simplistic explanation, it is not true in most color flow systems. In reality, the lines of color flow data are alternated with lines of anatomic scan data. The anatomic data are acquired and received by conventional means and the color flow data are acquired, received, and processed separately.

MULTIGATE DOPPLER

Doppler color flow instruments are all currently based upon pulsed wave (PW) Doppler methods. Conventional PW techniques are range gated. The Doppler sample volume is determined in range by the time it takes for the ultrasound pulse to travel to the area of interest and then back. If the same method was employed in color flow, it would simply take too long to sample over the entire image and there would be serious compromises made in frame rate.

Instead, all color flow systems are "multigated". This multigating takes advantage of Doppler information all along the line that is "ignored" in the conventional range-gated approach. In reality, each line has many gates that number in the hundreds.

It is best to think of the color flow map image as comprising little gates throughout the field of view, each gate containing some composite of the Doppler information. A typical image can consist of as many as 256 lines depending upon sector size and depth of range.

MORE ABOUT COLOR

All Doppler flow imaging systems encode the directions of flow into two primary colors: red and blue. Any number of color assignments could be made, but red and blue are chosen because they are primary colors of light (together with green).

Here is also relative flow velocity information in the color hues; the brighter the color the higher the velocity detected. Thus, high velocities away from the transducer will appear as lighter shades of blue, and higher velocities toward the

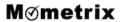

transducer will be represented by lighter shades of red, or even yellow. Low velocity flow will be represented by darker shades of these colors. Absence of flow is always represented by black.

Points of Discussion

RELATIONSHIP BETWEEN ULTRASOUND FREQUENCY AND DEPTH OF PENETRATION

Ultrasound frequency is the number of cycles or waves of sound per second and is measured in Megahertz (MHz) or million hertz range. Higher frequency ultrasound provides greater detail, but has poorer penetration of tissues. This is because the small wavelengths allow for the differentiation of very small structures. Lower frequency ultrasound provides less detail but does have better penetration of tissues.

Medical ultrasound frequencies range from 3.5 to 7.5 MHz. For deep structures 3.5 MHz is appropriate. This is the frequency that is used the most for ER scans including the abdominal trauma exam. For thin patients and children, 5 MHz may be used which will provide more detail than 3.5 MHz as depth of penetration is not as important. 5 MHz is useful for testicular scans and transvaginal exams where detail is more important than depth of penetration. Frequencies of 7.5 MHz have a few specific uses. The high frequency gives great detail, but the depth of penetration is poor. 7.5 MHz is used primarily for foreign bodies, testicular, transvaginal and vascular scans since these are modalities where fine detail is more important than penetration depth.

RELATIONSHIP BETWEEN ECHOGENICITY AND THE DEPICTION OF ULTRASOUND IMAGES AS WHITE, GRAY AND BLACK

Echogenicity refers to the ability of a substance to reflect or transmit ultrasound waves.

An echogenic image is an image that is produced by an object that reflects most ultrasound waves. It will appear white on the ultrasound screen.

An anechoic image is one that is produced by an object that transmits most ultrasound waves. It will appear dark or black on the ultrasound screen.

An image that is gray is produced by an object that both reflects and transmits ultrasound waves to varying degrees.

DIFFERENCE BETWEEN A MECHANICAL SECTOR SCANNER AND A LINEAR ELECTRONIC TRANSDUCER

In general, ultrasound devices all utilize a transducer. The transducer directs a narrow ultrasound beam along its line of sight, which returns a reflected ultrasound wave. This provides a one-dimensional line of information. By rapidly sweeping this line back and forth across a sector of tissue, a two-dimensional plane of information is generated, i.e., a cross-sectional ultrasound image of the tissue in question.

Mechanical sector scanners employ this principle by utilizing a small transducer element, which by rapidly pivoting back and forth (or through the use of a pivoting mirror), swings the ultrasound beam and generates a pie-shaped two-dimensional image. Since a single, small element is employed, these transducers are useful in situations where a narrow window is available, ie, imaging the heart through the space between two ribs.

As opposed to a singles winging beam, linear electronic (array) transducers utilize a linear arrangement (or array) of many small elements. When this device is held against the skin the elements fire rapidly in succession and in this fashion, generate a rectangular shaped two-dimensional image. Since many elements are required, linear arrays are longer (and more expensive) than mechanical sector scanners. In certain situations, this can be a disadvantage. The advantage of linear arrays, however, lies in the fact that by providing small alterations in the sequence of firing of the individual elements, changes in the direction and depth of focus of the beam can be instantaneously achieved.

CONVENTIONAL POSITION OF THE MARKER ON THE TRANSDUCER WHEN SCANNING IN THE CROSS-SECTIONAL PLANE

The cross-sectional or transverse ultrasound image should by convention, display the patient's right side of the body on the left side of the viewing monitor. The transverse ultrasound image is displayed so that the transverse "slice" is being viewed from the perspective of the patient's feet. (This is the same convention used for displaying CT images).

To produce a transverse image following this convention, the physician performing the exam should be on the patient's right side, and the transducer should be oriented in the transverse plane. The marker on the transducer should be directed towards the patient's right side. The resulting image will show a transverse view with the patient's right-sided structures (ie liver) on the left side of the monitor.

GAIN AND TGC (TIME GAIN COMPENSATOR)

GAIN refers to the amplification of the received signal. It is the artificial increase in the strength of the signal. All parts of the image on the screen are equally affected (as opposed to TGC). Adjustments of gain should be done with respect to tissues of known echogenicity.

The TGC (Time Gain Compensator) allows for 'fine tuning' of the attenuated signal. It allows one to sharpen the images of deeper is used when it is perceived that the gain in one part of the field is unequal to that of another.

COMMON ULTRASOUND ARTIFACTS

PSEUDO-SLUDGE (BEAM-WIDTH ARTIFACT)

When the focal zone of the transducer is at the center of the gallbladder, the beam is of greater width at the posterior border of the gallbladder. The partial volume effect along the posterior wall results in the appearance of sludge (but it is really the posterior gallbladder wall). Also, gas bubbles in the duodenum can be projected adjacent to the gallbladder, simulating a gallstone.

SIDE LOBE ARTIFACT

This artifact is caused when weaker sound beams from the sides of the transducer are returned by a very reflective bowel-gas interface. This may appear as a line within the lumen of the gallbladder. To eliminate this artifact, try and alternate the angle of the transducer head.

REVERBERATION ARTIFACT

This artifact is caused when ultrasound waves are being bounced back and forth between two or more highly reflective surfaces such as in the abdominal wall or a foreign body.

MIRROR EFFECT

Mirror effect is caused when the ultrasound beam is reflected back into the liver by the diaphragm and bounces back again to the transducer via the diaphragm. This results in intrahepatic structures appearing as if cephalad to the diaphragm.

GAIN ARTIFACTS

Gain artifacts are caused by both overuse of gain in an attempt to enhance structures or under use of gain, which results in eliminating tissue character.

CONTACT ARTIFACT

When insufficient gel is used, the transducer makes only intermittent contact with the skin surface resulting in contact artifact.

6 INTENSITIES

Putting together spatial and temporal considerations we end up with 6 intensities:

- Spatial average-temporal average (SATA)
- Spatial peak-temporal average (SPTA)
- Spatial average-pulse average (SAPA)
- Spatial peak-pulse average (SPPA)
- Spatial average-temporal peak (SATP)
- Spatial peak-temporal peak (SPTP)

Since SATA averages both in space and time it's the lowest value. SPTP does not average --> highest value.

TIS/TIB/TIC

The **Soft Tissue Thermal Index (TIS)** is meant to be displayed for examinations in which the ultrasound beam travels a path which is made up principally of homogeneous soft tissue or a soft tissue/fluid path, as in a first trimester fetal examination or an abdominal examination. The **Bone Thermal Index (TIB)** is applicable to examinations in which bone is exposed to ultrasound, as could occur during Doppler blood flow examinations of a second or third trimester fetus. The **Cranial Bone Thermal Index (TIC)** pertains to examinations in which bone is at or very near the surface of the transducer, such as during transcranial, Doppler blood flow examinations.

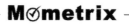

ALARA principle of ultrasound exposure: **A**s **L**ow **A**s **R**easonably **A**chievable.

Key Organizations

American Institute of Ultrasound in Medicine

http://www.aium.org/

National Electrical Manufacturers Association

http://www.nema.org/

Key Exam Facts

- Ultrasound velocity is greatest in bone 4000 m/sec blood and muscle is about 1570 m/sec while fat is the slowest at about 1450 m/sec.
- The length of the fresnel zone increases when radius of transducer increases.
- Reverberation artifacts are caused by multiple reflections from interfaces.
- Doppler imaging in ultrasound detects change in frequency of sound.
- Speed of sound in a medium depends on the density of medium.
- Concerning Doppler studies change in frequency is related to blood flow.
- decibels are attenuated per cm for ultrasound in soft tissue.
- The amount of reflection at an interface is due to differences in acoustical impedance, and angle of incidence.
- Axial resolution (size in mm) in ultrasound is directly proportional to pulse length and constant with depth.
- Non specular reflections are those involving objects which are smaller than the ultrasound beam. The generally give weak signal since only a portion of the beam is reflected back towards transducer
- Concerning the thickness of the transducer used in ultrasound resonance occurs when the thickness is equal to 1/2 wavelength
- Q factor is calculated as operating frequency/bandwidth bandwidth is the range of frequency produces. We want the bandwidth to be small (i.e., a 3MHz transducer should only produce 3MHz sound). The more of other frequencies that are produced the lower the Q factor. The pure 3MHz is degraded.
- Lateral resolution depends upon the number of scan lines and the width of the ultrasound beam
- When a piezo electric crystal in an ultrasound transducer has a negative voltage induced in it, this is caused by dipoles.
- The TGC control in ultrasound compensates for differences in acoustical impedance.
- Aliasing in real-time ultrasound may be reduced by increasing the number of scan lines.
- The TGC is used in ultrasound to increase amplification of echoes at increased depths.
- A 5 MHz ultrasound beam passes from soft tissue to bone intensity is reduced significantly.
- Axial resolution in ultrasound is generally better than lateral resolution.
- Reverberation artifacts are caused by multiple reflections of same interface.
- The thickness of the transducer used in ultrasound are determined by thickness equal to 1/2 wavelength.
- Acoustic shadowing results when an ultrasound beam strikes a high attenuation.

- The amount of doppler shift is effect by turbulence, stenosis, and peak systolic.
- The lateral resolution in Ultrasound Imaging is determined by Beam Focusing and number of scan lines.
- The Doppler frequency increases when velocity increases, and greater transducer frequency.
- The critical angle in US refers to the angle at which all incident intensity is reflected.
- The 1/4 matching layer in ultrasound is used to increase the transmitted intensity into the patient.
- The following formula can be used to calculate Incident Beam after attenuation:
- $dB = 10 \log I_1 / I_2$

ARDMS Practice Test

1. Sonographers should be aware of work-related musculoskeletal disorders. Best practice while scanning is to avoid abducting the arm more than how many degrees?

    a. 50
    b. 90
    c. 30
    d. 40

2. Which action demonstrates best practice during ultrasound exams regarding the ALARA principle?

    a. The exposure time should be extended during the exam.
    b. Use the lowest possible output power that provides a diagnostic image.
    c. Use the lowest possible gain.
    d. Ensure that the time gain compensation (TGC) is within acceptable limits.

3. Which type of cavitation is the MOST concerning cause of bioeffects?

    a. Transient
    b. Absorption
    c. Stable
    d. Thermal

4. Assuming an unfocused ultrasound beam, the American Institute of Ultrasound in Medicine's "Statement on Mammalian Biological Effects of Ultrasound In Vivo" has confirmed that no bioeffects have been noted when the spatial pulse temporal average (SPTA) intensity is less than which value?

    a. 1 mW/cm^2
    b. 100 W/cm^2
    c. 1 W/cm^2
    d. 100 mW/cm^2

5. A sonographer notices that the mechanical index (MI) is too high during an ultrasound. What would be the MOST appropriate modification that the sonographer can make?

    a. Decrease receiver gain.
    b. Increase period.
    c. Decrease the output power.
    d. Decrease the frequency of the transducer.

6. Select the technique that will generate the LEAST amount of exposure to the patient.

    a. Spectral Doppler
    b. Color flow Doppler
    c. Grayscale
    d. M-mode

7. When a vibrating string or fluid pump is used to test system performance, what parameter is being tested?

    a. Dead zone
    b. Doppler velocities
    c. Contrast resolution
    d. Grayscale sensitivity

8. A tissue-equivalent phantom is used to ensure the efficiency of the ultrasound machine. Choose the resolution that is NOT tested with this phantom.

    a. Temporal
    b. Contrast
    c. Axial
    d. Horizontal

9. Which performance check describes the ability of the ultrasound machine to correctly visualize signals that are weaker than others?

    a. Accuracy
    b. Specificity
    c. Reliability
    d. Sensitivity

10. What is the name of the recent technological advancement that is used on tissues such as the liver, breast, prostate, and thyroid to assess the stiffness of tissue or to better assess lesions?

    a. Contrast-enhanced ultrasound
    b. Fusion imaging
    c. Elastography
    d. Harmonics

11. Which choice is NOT a true statement regarding this filling defect within the gallbladder?

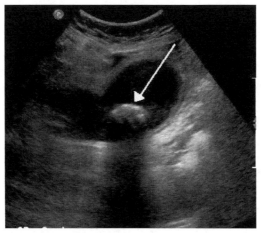

   a. The filling defect displays a significant amount of attenuation.
   b. It has created an enhancement artifact.
   c. It has created a shadowing artifact.
   d. Regions deeper than the filling defect are obscured.

12. Which type of artifact appears echogenic and stems from gas bubbles as they vibrate due to the interaction with the ultrasound beam?
   a. Ring-down artifact
   b. Edge shadow
   c. Crosstalk
   d. Slice thickness

13. What is the fundamental reason that the power and intensity of the ultrasound beam diminish as it travels through tissue?
   a. Absorption
   b. Cavitation
   c. Obstruction
   d. Acoustic impedance

14. Select the modification that the sonographer can make to decrease the amount of attenuation as the ultrasound beam travels through tissues.
   a. Increase the imaging depth.
   b. Increase the frequency of the transducer.
   c. Decrease the output power.
   d. Decrease the frequency of the transducer.

15. Choose the ultrasound system function that enables the sonographer to adapt to the amount of attenuation that occurs with increasing depth.

a. Focusing
b. Receiver gain
c. TGC
d. Output power

16. Assume that a sound beam is traveling in soft tissue. Calculate the attenuation coefficient if the frequency is 12 MHz.

a. 12 dB/cm
b. 6 dB/cm
c. 8 dB/cm
d. 10 dB/cm

17. What is NOT a component of attenuation?

a. Reflection
b. Scattering
c. Resolution
d. Absorption

18. Impedance is NOT influenced by which component?

a. The frequency of the transducer
b. Density
c. Propagation speed
d. Stiffness

19. For reflection to take place, which situation must exist?

a. The border of two different tissues must have different impedances.
b. There must be little difference of the impedances at soft-tissue boundaries.
c. Normal incidence and identical impedances must be present.
d. Oblique incidence must occur.

20. While assuming continuous wave (CW) ultrasound, what is the duty factor (DF)?

a. 0.2%
b. 1%
c. 0%
d. 100%

21. What will happen to the duty factor (DF) if the system increases the pulse repetition frequency (PRF)?

a. DF remains the same.
b. DF increases.
c. DF is not related to PRF.
d. DF decreases.

22. The best axial resolution will be apparent if the sonographer performs an exam with a transducer that has which characteristic?

    a. Longer pulse length
    b. Longer wavelength
    c. Shorter pulse length
    d. More ringing in the pulse

23. Lateral resolution will be improved if the sonographer performs which operation?

    a. Decreases the scanning depth
    b. Increases the number of focal zones
    c. Maximizes the output power
    d. Uses a lower frequency

24. Which action will NOT increase (or improve) temporal resolution?

    a. Increase the imaging depth.
    b. Decrease the number of focal zones.
    c. Use a sector size that is narrow.
    d. Use a low line density.

25. Which name describes how the angles of the incident and transmission beams are related to the speed of the two media?

    a. Bernoulli's principle
    b. Curie point
    c. Huygens' principle
    d. Snell's law

26. What can be done when investigating a possible kidney stone to better demonstrate shadowing from the stone when using a 3 MHz probe?

    a. Position the focal point deeper than the stone.
    b. Increase the amount of gain.
    c. Increase the frequency to 5 MHz.
    d. Decrease the output power of the system.

27. If the frequency is doubled, what effect will this have on the wavelength?

    a. It will remain the same.
    b. It doubles.
    c. It increases by a factor of 1.54.
    d. It is halved.

28. Which part of the transducer is necessary to reduce the amount of ringing of the piezoelectric (PZT) crystal?

    a. Matching layer
    b. Backing material
    c. Transducer housing
    d. Wire

29. A given frequency of sound is 4.5 MHz, and it has a wavelength of 0.8 mm. How thick should a manufacturer design the matching layer of a transducer in this scenario?

    a. 0.4 mm
    b. 0.16 mm
    c. 0.2 mm
    d. 0.6 mm

30. A sonographer is performing a renal ultrasound. Which transducer frequency will generate the slowest speed of sound?

    a. All frequencies will travel at the same speed in the same tissue.
    b. 2 MHz
    c. 4.5 MHz
    d. 7 MHz

31. Transducers used in image production will have which characteristics?

    a. High Q-factor, wide bandwidth
    b. Low Q-factor, wide bandwidth
    c. Low Q-factor, narrow bandwidth
    d. High Q-factor, narrow bandwidth

32. Which transducer produced the shape of this image?

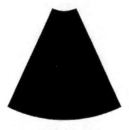

    a. Linear sequential array
    b. Vector array
    c. Annular phased array
    d. Convex array

33. This malfunction takes place in which kind of transducer?

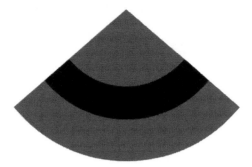

   a. Linear sequential array
   b. Annular phased array
   c. Convex sequential array
   d. Mechanical

34. Which statement is NOT true of a linear phased array transducer?

   a. The footprint tends to be small.
   b. It can alter the number of focal zones and the depth.
   c. The image is a rectangle.
   d. It uses electronic steering.

35. Select the type of transducer that enables multi-focusing while being steered mechanically.

   a. Annular phased array
   b. Mechanical
   c. Linear sequential array
   d. Convex sequential array

36. If the diameter of the PZT crystal is 13 mm, which sentence describes the sound wave's diameter in the Fresnel zone?

   a. The sound beam will be half of the diameter of the crystal in the Fresnel zone.
   b. 13 mm
   c. 26 mm
   d. The sound wave narrows as it leaves the transducer.

37. The amount of divergence that occurs in the far field is determined by the sound wave's frequency and which component?

   a. Line density
   b. Focal zone depth
   c. Diameter of the crystal
   d. Speed

38. Select the type of transducer that produces an image that takes on the shape of a parallelogram when it is electronically steered.

    a. Linear phased array
    b. Linear sequential array
    c. Annular phased array
    d. Convex array

39. Choose the type of transducer that lacks range resolution.

    a. Phased array
    b. Annular array
    c. Continuous wave (CW)
    d. Linear sequential array

40. In this phased array transducer, what direction will the beam be steered?

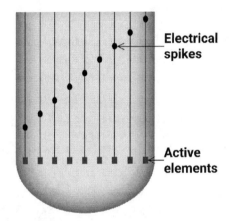

    a. 45 degrees to the right
    b. Slightly to the left
    c. Slightly to the right
    d. 45 degrees to the left

41. What configuration is necessary to focus the ultrasound wave in a linear phased array transducer?

    a. Electronic slope
    b. Dynamic aperture
    c. PZT crystals
    d. Electronic curve

42. Which parameter is decreased by the ultrasound machine to evade the possibility of range ambiguity when the imaging depth is increased?

    a. Number of scan lines
    b. Pulse repetition frequency (PRF)
    c. Pulse repetition period (PRP)
    d. Persistence

43. Which phrase does NOT describe an effect that focusing has on the ultrasound beam?

    a. A bigger focal zone
    b. Enhanced near zone resolution
    c. Diminished lateral resolution of the far zone
    d. Results in a shorter near zone

44. Select the answer that best describes how B-mode will typically display blood vessels?

    a. Hyperechoic
    b. Isogenic
    c. Anechoic
    d. Heterogeneous

45. How deep is a reflector if the go-return time of a sound wave is 39 μs?

    a. 2 cm
    b. 3 cm
    c. 5 cm
    d. 6 cm

46. Why does grayscale imaging require the use of pulsed wave ultrasound?

    a. To optimize penetration
    b. To optimize temporal resolution
    c. To determine the bandwidth
    d. To determine the depth of the reflector

47. Which system function is modified if the ultrasound user adjusts the receiver gain?

    a. Demodulation
    b. Reject
    c. Amplification
    d. Compression

48. When M-mode is employed during an echocardiogram, what information is depicted on the display?

    a. Depth and amplitude
    b. Time and frequency
    c. Amplitude, motion, and time
    d. Depth, time, and frequency

49. If an ultrasound image displays high contrast, what correlates with the dynamic range?

    a. Wide dynamic range
    b. Narrow dynamic range
    c. No effect on the range
    d. A display of many shades of gray

50. Which component of the ultrasound wave increases if the sonographer increases the output gain?

a. Pulse duration
b. Frequency
c. Noise
d. Intensity

51. What is the name of the frequency used in tissue harmonics that is responsible for image production?

a. Fundamental frequency
b. Spatial compounding
c. Overall gain
d. Harmonic frequency

52. Which one of the following applies when using tissue harmonics to image the gallbladder?

a. Use of lower frequencies
b. Use of higher frequencies
c. Decreased lateral resolution
d. Increased reverberation artifacts

53. Which type of zoom is a preprocessing function that provides more pixels in the region of interest, resulting in superior spatial resolution?

a. Temporal resolution
b. Read zoom
c. Write zoom
d. Read magnification

54. Which control on the ultrasound system should be adjusted if it is necessary to reduce the amount of noise in the image?

a. Reject
b. Amplification
c. Compression
d. Demodulation

55. During a renal ultrasound, the sonographer finds it necessary to adjust controls on the ultrasound system to improve the image. What CANNOT be adjusted by the operator?

a. Output power
b. Amplitude
c. Frequency
d. Speed

56. What control offers better visualization of fibroids by increasing far field penetration and resolution?

    a. Persistence
    b. Spatial compounding
    c. Coded excitation
    d. Elastography

57. Which control can a sonographer apply to help delineate a subtle liver mass?

    a. Zoom
    b. Edge enhancement
    c. Fill-in interpolation
    d. Increase the receiver gain

58. Which phrase correctly describes the following ultrasound beam?

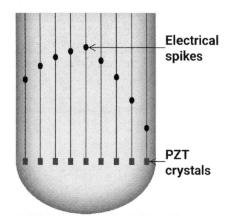

    a. Unfocused, no steering
    b. Focused, steered to the right
    c. Unfocused, steered to the left
    d. Focused, steered to the left

59. What is the name of the approach to image production in which the reflected ultrasound beam is averaged among multiple frequencies to lessen the effects of noise and speckle in the image?

    a. Spatial compounding
    b. Tissue harmonics
    c. Frequency compounding
    d. Temporal compounding

60. What is a function of the receiver?

    a. It shapes the ultrasound beam.
    b. It controls the collaboration of the synergy of the ultrasound components.
    c. It stores images and video clips.
    d. It changes and displays the signal sent from the transducer to the monitor.

61. What is the correct order in which the receiver functions during image production?

a. Amplification, compensation, compression, demodulation, reject
b. Amplification, reject, demodulation, compensation, compression
c. Amplification, demodulation, compression, reject, compensation
d. Amplification, compression, demodulation, reject, compensation

62. Preprocessing functions occur before the data reaches which component of the ultrasound system?

a. Pulser
b. Scan converter
c. Receiver
d. Beam former

63. Which phrase describes the scenario in which persistence will be best used?

a. When persistence cannot be adjusted by the user
b. During the interrogation of rapid blood flow
c. During the interrogation of slow blood flow
d. When more noise is desired during image production

64. When using 3D ultrasound, what is the name of the smallest element of the picture that is generated?

a. Pixel
b. Voxel
c. Byte
d. Bit

65. Digital imaging systems require which component to link the ultrasound system and the archiving network?

a. BIT
b. RIS
c. PACS
d. DICOM

66. Which component enables facilities that use digital imaging to archive and share the images of exams performed in the department?

a. RIS
b. PACS
c. BIT
d. DICOM

67. Which list describes the progression in which a signal moves through an ultrasound machine?

    a. Scan converter, transducer, display, receiver
    b. Transducer, scan converter, display, receiver
    c. Scan converter, receiver, display, transducer
    d. Transducer, receiver, scan converter, display

68. Which choice will optimize the spatial resolution?

    a. $1,500 \times 1,500$ analog
    b. 200×200 pixels
    c. 800×800 pixels
    d. 300×300 digital

69. Which system control was used to create the following image?

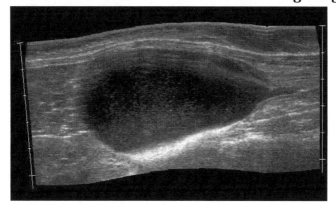

    a. Elastography
    b. Color Doppler
    c. Extended field of view (EFOV)
    d. B-mode

70. Which region is NOT a component of a TGC curve?

    a. Phase quadrature
    b. Knee
    c. Near gain
    d. Slope

71. If 3 bits of memory are available, what is the greatest number of shades of gray that are present in the scan converter?

    a. 4
    b. 8
    c. 16
    d. 32

72. The best contrast resolution will be available with which digital scan converter?

    a. 4 bits
    b. 256 shades of gray
    c. 32 shades of gray
    d. 16 bits

73. Which scanning angles will provide the most significant amount of Doppler shift to measure the peak velocity during a carotid duplex ultrasound?

    a. 0 or 90 degrees
    b. 90 or 180 degrees
    c. 115 or 180 degrees
    d. 0 or 180 degrees

74. Which image demonstrates the correct placement of the gate to obtain the most accurate blood flow velocity measurement?

a.

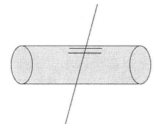

b.

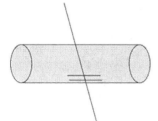

c.

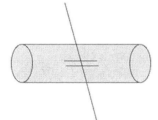

d.

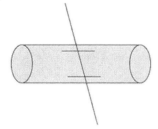

75. Which of the following represents the approximate diameter reduction of the internal carotid artery (ICA) when evaluating the spectral waveform and peak systolic velocity (PSV) and end-diastolic velocity (EDV) information?

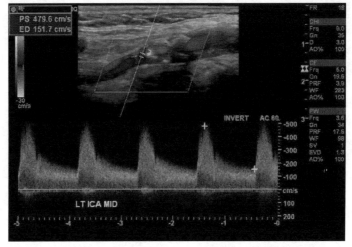

a. 25–49%
b. 50–79%
c. 80–99%
d. 100%

76. If a sonographer asks a patient to take in a deep breath and hold it, what is the result of venous blood flow in the legs?

a. The flow becomes turbulent.
b. The flow rate decreases.
c. The flow rate increases.
d. The flow becomes pulsatile.

77. Which statement is true regarding these images?

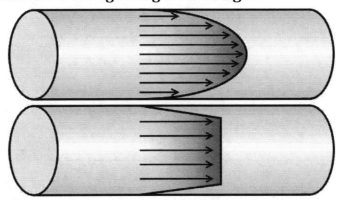

a. The blood flow represented in these vessels is considered to be laminar flow.
b. The Reynolds number in these vessels is likely more than 2,000.
c. The blood flow represented in these vessels will be chaotic.
d. Eddy currents will likely be present within these blood vessels.

78. If a carotid duplex exam is performed on a patient with a 7 MHz and a 14 MHz transducer, which transducer will display a Doppler shift that is greater?

    a. The 14 MHz transducer

    b. The Doppler shift is the same with both transducers.

    c. The 7 MHz transducer

    d. The Doppler shift cannot be identified with this information.

79. Which step CANNOT be used to correct the imaging error seen in the following tracing of the external carotid artery (ECA)?

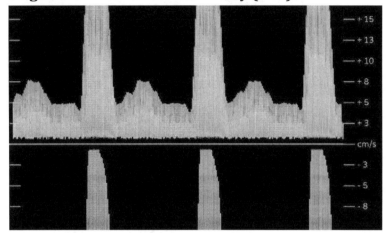

    a. Switch to a lower frequency transducer.

    b. Move the baseline down.

    c. Reposition the gate to a location that is deeper.

    d. Increase the pulse repetition frequency (PRF) to its maximum value.

80. While using pulsed wave Doppler, the sonographer believes that the measurements are not accurate. After switching to a 4.5 MHz continuous wave (CW) Doppler at a depth of 5 cm, what will the maximum velocity cap be?

    a. There will not be a maximum velocity cap with CW Doppler.

    b. 45 cm/s

    c. 150 cm/s

    d. This cannot be determined with the given information.

81. What will the aliasing frequency be if a renal artery duplex exam is performed at a depth of 6 cm, the length of the sample volume is 0.50 mm, and the pulse repetition frequency (PRF) is 8 kHz with the Doppler frequency at 3.5 MHz?

    a. 3.5 MHz

    b. 8 kHz

    c. 7 MHz

    d. 4 kHz

82. Which statement is NOT true concerning color Doppler?

a. Doppler frequency shift is reached with the use of the autocorrelation method.
b. Aliasing may occur when using color Doppler.
c. Color Doppler is a reliable method to measure the peak systolic and end-diastolic velocities.
d. Range resolution exists with color Doppler.

83. If a sonographer must interrogate a blood vessel that displays slow flow once color Doppler is applied, what should be done to the pulse repetition frequency (PRF) to improve the visualization of flow?

a. Adjusting the PRF has no effect.
b. Decrease the PRF.
c. Increase the PRF.
d. Adjusting the PRF will create aliasing.

84. If the red blood cells are traveling away from the transducer, what type of Doppler shift is present?

a. Negative
b. Unequivocal
c. None
d. Positive

85. A sonographer has access to 10 MHz linear sequential, 7 MHz linear sequential, and 4.5 MHz curved array transducers. If the 10 MHz transducer produces aliasing during a carotid duplex study, what can be done to alleviate this issue if a shallower window did NOT correct the problem?

a. Switch to the 4.5 MHz curved array transducer.
b. Neither of the two remaining transducers will resolve this issue.
c. Switch to the 7 MHz linear sequential transducer.
d. None of these transducers should be used for carotid duplex exams.

86. If the sonographer does not see any color flow when applied but could see movement of blood cells within the vessel on grayscale imaging, what should the operator assume?

a. Power Doppler must be used instead.
b. The angle of incidence is 90 degrees and needs to be changed.
c. The blood vessel is obstructed.
d. Maintenance must be called as the color Doppler is not sensitive enough.

87. When using spectral Doppler, the sonographer notices information that correlates with lower velocities missing from the waveform. What control can be modified to demonstrate these velocities?

    a. Wall filter
    b. Scale
    c. Depth
    d. Gain

88. If the Reynolds number is 2,078, what does this suggest?

    a. Plug flow
    b. Laminar flow
    c. Disturbed flow
    d. Turbulent flow

89. The carotid artery is being examined with color Doppler. Which artifact is present if the color appears to be bleeding outside of the vessel when color Doppler is applied?

    a. Clutter
    b. Crosstalk
    c. Ghosting
    d. Aliasing

90. If a sonographer measures the peak systolic velocity (PSV) from the ICA and the spectral window appears filled in with blood moving in various directions, what does this indicate?

    a. Spectral broadening
    b. Patent ICA
    c. The gain is set too high.
    d. Laminar flow

91. The ultrasound operator is attempting to measure the velocity of flow within the femoral artery but is incidentally picking up signals within the femoral vein. Which control on the ultrasound system will enable the sonographer to adjust the position of the gate?

    a. Angle correction
    b. Triplex
    c. Sweep speed
    d. Pulse repetition frequency (PRF)

92. If it is necessary to improve the frame rate during a color Doppler exam, which step is the best action to accomplish this?

    a. Angle the color box.
    b. Decrease the gain.
    c. Increase the depth in which the color box is located.
    d. Decrease the width of the color box.

93. Which operator setting will increase the patient's exposure during a carotid duplex exam?

   a. Increasing the Doppler angle
   b. Increasing the pulse repetition frequency (PRF)
   c. A higher baseline location
   d. Increasing the Doppler gain

94. Which operation will improve the frame rate when using color Doppler to interrogate the ovaries?

   a. Change the color map.
   b. Increase the packet size.
   c. Decrease the packet size.
   d. Adjust the color Doppler gain.

95. Which is NOT a reason a sonographer would choose to use power Doppler during a renal duplex exam?

   a. The velocity of the blood is accurately measured with power Doppler.
   b. Aliasing will not occur with power Doppler.
   c. The sensitivity of power Doppler is greater than that of color Doppler.
   d. The amplitude of the signal is displayed with power Doppler.

96. Aliasing is seen while scanning the femoral artery at a 30-degree angle. Which step will correct this artifact?

   a. Reduce the angle of incidence.
   b. Increase the frequency of the transducer.
   c. Find a window that is deeper.
   d. Increase the pulse repetition frequency (PRF).

97. A sonographer uses the color map during a color Doppler exam of the carotid artery and notices that the colors in the middle of the map appear to be communicating with each other. Which choice best describes this scenario?

   a. Aliasing is present.
   b. The flow in the carotid artery is bidirectional.
   c. The flow in the carotid artery is unidirectional.
   d. The wall filter is set too high.

98. When the screen is sector shaped, what can be modified when color Doppler is used?

   a. Steering of the color box
   b. Size and location of the color box
   c. Shape of the color box
   d. Velocity of the moving red blood cells

99. Which choice will improve the color fill of this blood vessel?

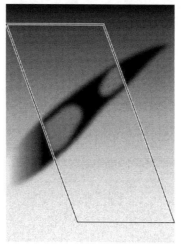

a. Change the steering of the color box.
b. Increase the output power.
c. Change the window so the vessel is shallower.
d. Decrease the color gain.

100. Which choice is NOT an instance of when a sonographer would expect to see spectral broadening?

a. When sampling the velocity within a tight stenosis of the internal carotid artery
b. When sampling the velocity distal to a tight stenosis of the external carotid artery
c. When measuring the velocity within a patent internal carotid artery
d. When sampling the velocity at the bifurcation of the carotid artery

Answer Key and Explanations

1. C: Sonographers should use correct ergonomics to care for their own bodies to prevent work-related musculoskeletal disorders. Roughly 80% of sonographers report having some sort of work injury. Ergonomics is a combination of setting up the room appropriately so the patient and machine can be reached easily. Properly using equipment that reinforces the desired body mechanics to prevent any injuries is also key. This may be something as simple as adjusting the keyboard or monitor to the correct height. One of the most common complaints that a sonographer makes is pain in the shoulder while scanning. It is imperative that the patient is close enough so that the sonographer's arm does not have to be abducted more than 30 degrees. The other choices would not protect the sonographer because they are all angles that are more than 30 degrees.

2. B: Sonographers should always consider ways to practice the ALARA principle. ALARA stands for as low as reasonably achievable, and sonographers can achieve this by using the lowest possible output power that enables a diagnostic image. Keeping the exposure time to a minimum is another effective way of practicing ALARA. The gain can change the brightness (or darkness) of the image, but it has no effect on patient exposure, so the power should always be reduced, if possible, before the gain to reduce exposure to the patient. On the other hand, if an image is too dark, it is best to increase the gain because it will not affect exposure to the patient. Time gain compensation (TGC) enables the sonographer to adjust the amplification of reflections that are located at a greater depth in the body, but it has no effect on the exposure.

3. A: Cavitation is discussed when bioeffects are considered with the interaction of the ultrasound beam and gas bubbles in the human body. Higher temperatures and pressures may cause the gas bubbles within the body to burst; this is known as transient cavitation, which is extremely concerning for harmful bioeffects. When these gas bubbles expand and contract with fluctuations in pressure without rupturing, it is referred to as stable cavitation. There are only two types of cavitation, so absorption and thermal are not viable answers to this question.

4. D: The spatial pulse temporal average (SPTA) is linked with the greatest amount of temperature elevation within tissues. Bioeffects have not been noted when the SPTA intensity was less than 100 mW/cm^2, when the ultrasound beam was unfocused. If the ultrasound beam is focused, then the same principle applies if the intensity is less than 1 W/cm^2. If there is an inquiry regarding the smallest intensity, the answer would be the spatial average temporal average.

5. C: The mechanical index (MI) is a parameter that the user should monitor to help determine if cavitation is expected. If a sonographer notices that the MI is too high during an ultrasound, it is important to decrease the acoustic power of the machine. Another step the sonographer can do to keep the MI lower is to *increase* the frequency of the transducer. The receiver gain has no effect on patient exposure.

116

The ultrasound operator is not able to adjust the period unless a different transducer is chosen.

6. C: The lowest level of tissue heating occurs when the output intensity of the equipment being used is at its lowest numerical value. Generally, grayscale imaging is the method in which tissue heating will be the lowest. It is typically the highest when pulsed Doppler is being used. M-mode and color flow Doppler tend to fall in the middle of these intensities.

Ultrasound should be used only for clinical exams in which the benefits outweigh the risks. One risk during an exam is an elevation of temperature in tissues exposed to the ultrasound beam. The thermal index (TI) will be highest during an exam with a high-frequency, high-intensity beam. This heating depends on the exposure time and the temperature. Typically, the greatest increase in temperature is witnessed with spectral Doppler exams.

7. B: A vibrating string or fluid pump is used to test Doppler velocities of an ultrasound system. These Doppler phantoms enable the evaluation of particles in motion that mimic blood flowing through blood vessels to determine the accuracy of velocities as well as the resolution at various depths. The dead zone is the region within the first centimeter of the transducer. Contrast resolution and grayscale sensitivity can both be evaluated with a tissue-equivalent phantom.

8. A: A tissue-equivalent phantom (also referred to as a grayscale or tissue-mimicking phantom) is important because it evaluates the sensitivity of the system's grayscale capabilities. This type of phantom can distinguish between shades of gray that are even marginally different, such as in contrast resolution. Axial resolution can also be evaluated with a tissue-equivalent phantom because separate structures that are parallel to the ultrasound wave can be seen individually as one in front of the other. Horizontal resolution is the ability to determine that reflectors are in the proper locations when they are perpendicular and in a horizontal position in relation to the ultrasound beam. Horizontal resolution can also be assessed in a tissue-equivalent phantom. Temporal resolution depends on the frame rate and is not tested with a tissue-equivalent phantom.

9. D: Sensitivity refers to the ability of an ultrasound machine to demonstrate weaker signals. Accuracy is the ability of an exam to diagnose outcomes that are positive and negative. Specificity is when an imaging exam can correctly diagnose results that are normal. Reliability refers to the ability of an exam to produce results that are dependable and consistent.

10. C: Elastography is a recent ultrasound technology that uses sound waves to test the stiffness of tissue or lesions that are being evaluated. Elastography is used most often when evaluating the liver, breast, or prostate or for thyroid disease. Contrast-enhanced ultrasound involves injecting (or giving orally) contrast to help visualize tumors or to evaluate blood vessels. Fusion imaging involves concurrent ultrasound imaging with a previous computed tomography or magnetic resonance imaging scan on a split screen to enhance diagnostic confidence that an area previously mentioned is the same area being evaluated. This can be extremely helpful during ultrasound-guided biopsies. Harmonics are signals that are produced by the patient's body (not the ultrasound system). This technology has been in use for several years.

11. B: In this image, a gallstone (cholelithiasis) is the filling defect that is visualized within the lumen of the gallbladder. Artifacts can offer important information such as shadowing from something that is calcified such as a gallstone, as seen in this instance, or even a kidney stone. This filling defect attenuates a great deal and has created a shadowing artifact, which is the hypoechoic area that is seen underneath the gallstone. The regions deep to the filling defect are obscured due to the shadowing. The opposite of a shadowing artifact is one that is known as an enhancement artifact. This type of artifact can also be advantageous for sonographers and interpreting physicians because it appears as a hyperechoic region underneath a structure that demonstrates a lower attenuation rate such as a cyst or the gallbladder.

12. A: A ring-down artifact (also known as a comet-tail artifact) occurs when the reflectors are parallel to the ultrasound beam; it looks like an echogenic line. An edge shadow is due to the refraction of the sound beam; it appears like a dark shadow that extends deep to a curved structure. Crosstalk occurs only with spectral Doppler as a mirror image artifact in which blood flow looks as if it is moving in two directions. A slice-thickness artifact can degrade image details if the slice thickness of the ultrasound beam is wider than the target. When this takes place, fluid-filled components may not be visualized at all or they may look like they are filled in because the return signal is including soft tissue on either side of the cyst at the same depth.

13. A: Attenuation is a term that describes the weakening of the ultrasound beam as it passes through tissues. This weakening applies to the power, amplitude, and intensity of the beam. The fundamental cause of attenuation is absorption because the energy of the beam is changed to heat. Cavitation refers to the possibility of bioeffects occurring during an exam. Obstruction is not a term that is related to attenuation, and acoustic impedance is the hindrance of sound as it passes through a medium, which affects the reflection of a sound wave.

14. D: The amount of attenuation will be decreased if the sonographer decreases the frequency of the transducer. Absorption is one of the main causes of attenuation, and attenuation increases when the sonographer increases the frequency of the transducer, making this choice incorrect. The distance that the sound wave travels has a direct impact on attenuation, so increasing the imaging depth will increase attenuation (not decrease as asked in this instance). Decreasing the output power creates more attenuation because the ultrasound wave is not as strong.

15. C: Time gain compensation (TGC) is a function of the ultrasound system that allows the sonographer to compensate for the weaker signals (attenuation) as the sound waves travel further into the body. This control will allow for uniform brightness when set correctly because the user can adjust at specific depths when necessary. Receiver gain will implement a change to the entire image and not just at certain depths. Focusing will create a beam that is narrower at the focal point, enhancing the resolution at this point. Adjusting the output power will either increase or decrease the energy of the ultrasound beam, creating an entire image that is brighter or darker and affects patient exposure.

16. B: The attenuation coefficient describes how the intensity of the ultrasound beam decreases when considering the distance and frequency of the ultrasound wave. The attenuation coefficient units are decibels per centimeter (dB/cm). Attenuation occurs because of reflection, scattering, and absorption of the sound beam's energy. Frequency is directly related to scattering and absorption, so we can assume that frequency is also directly related to the attenuation coefficient. The equation that can be used to calculate this is as follows:

$$\text{Attenuation coefficient (dB/cm)} = \frac{\text{frequency (MHz)}}{2} = \frac{12}{2} = 6\,\text{dB/cm}.$$

17. C: Resolution refers to image quality and is not a component of attenuation. Recall that as a sound beam passes through the body, the intensity is diminished (as are the amplitude and power). Three components contribute to the attenuation of a sound beam: reflection, scattering, and absorption. Reflection occurs if a part of the sound beam is sent back toward the transducer. Specular and diffuse are two types of reflections. Specular reflection takes place when there is a smooth boundary such as looking in a mirror. This portion of the beam, however, does not return directly back to the transducer but at an angle. Diffuse reflections take place at a boundary that is not smooth and tends to reflect in various directions known as backscatter. Scattering is the second component of attenuation that occurs when the energy tends to travel in many directions. One cannot predict where scattering will take place, and an ultrasound beam with a higher frequency will demonstrate more scatter. Absorption is the third component of attenuation; it describes when the energy of the ultrasound wave is changed to heat.

18. A: Impedance can be defined as the interference of the transmission of sound as it moves through tissue. Impedance is the product of the medium's density and propagation speed of the medium, so if the density and speed increase, impedance will also increase. Acoustic impedance is a calculation that has an impact on the amount of reflection that occurs. If two tissues have the same impedance, all of the sound will be transmitted. If two tissue types have vastly different impedances, the majority of the sound will be reflected. Stiffness has a direct relationship to speed, therefore also influencing impedance. The frequency of the transducer does not influence the impedance because impedance is related only to the medium.

19. A: Reflection takes places when some of the energy of the sound wave is averted back toward the transducer. Reflection will occur only if the borders of two different tissues have different impedances; otherwise, transmission occurs. Recall that the incident intensity is the intensity of a sound beam as it leaves the transducer prior to coming into contact with tissue. The transmitted intensity is the forward propagation of the intensity of the incident beam after hitting that boundary. Normal incidence is when the incident sound beam comes into contact with the boundary at a 90-degree angle. During diagnostic imaging, there are few differences in the impedance of soft-tissue boundaries; therefore, more than 99% of the incident beam will be transmitted. To summarize, with normal incidence and identical impedances of the media, all of the incident beam's intensity will be transmitted. Keep in mind that the incident and transmitted intensities must always equal 100%. Oblique incidence and reflection (or transmission) are hard to conclude because they tend to be complex.

20. D: Duty factor (DF) is the percentage of time that an ultrasound system is imparting sound waves. For continuous wave (CW) systems, the DF is 100% because a signal is always being sent (but is unable to generate an ultrasound image because images can be created only with pulsed waves). A DF of 0% means that a system is not generating a pulse. Recall that the maximum value for DF of a CW sound beam is 100% and the minimum value is 0%. Pulses are necessary to create images, and the typical DF for imaging is 0.2%, which is for pulsed wave systems.

21. B: The DF is the percentage of time that a transducer is actively transmitting a signal. DF is a calculation that has no units; rather, it will be expressed as a percentage. The ranges of DF for clinical imaging fall into the 0.002–0.005 range or 0.2%–0.5%. These ranges of diagnostic ultrasound indicate that a small percentage of time is spent transmitting a pulse and a large percentage of time is used for listening. The DF is calculated by the following equation:

$$DF = \frac{\text{pulse duration}}{\text{pulse repetition period (PRP)}} \times 100.$$

The pulse repetition frequency (PRF) is defined as the number of pulses sent into the body in one second. DF and PRF are both affected by the imaging depth and will have a direct relationship with each other, which makes incorrect. The PRF is inversely related to the depth of the object being studied, as is the DF. As the depth decreases, the PRF increases because new pulses are constantly being sent because the listening time is shorter. If the depth increases, the PRF decreases (as will the DF) because there is more listening time, so the return time has to be greater. If the PRF increases, DF also increases because the amount of time the system is "on," or transmitting a pulse, increases.

22. C: Axial resolution is enhanced when shorter pulse lengths are being produced. Axial resolution is considered superior to lateral resolution in diagnostic imaging because ultrasound pulses tend to be shorter than the width of the beam. It should be noted that an increase in focusing tends to degrade axial resolution because the result is a longer pulse length. More ringing in the pulse indicates that more cycles are present in the pulse, and, therefore, the axial resolution will not be improved.

23. B: Lateral resolution depends on the width of the ultrasound beam. It will be improved if the sonographer increases the number of focal zones while scanning a patient because this is the narrowest portion of the beam (focus). Lateral resolution is enhanced at the focus. This action will, however, slow down the frame rate. Lateral resolution (also referred to as angular, azimuthal, and transverse) describes the capability of the system to demonstrate separate reflectors when they are perpendicular to the ultrasound beam. If the user decreases the scanning depth, this will improve the lateral resolution only when it is the focal point as well, but unlike axial resolution, the lateral resolution does change with the imaging depth. The output power will not affect the lateral resolution. Switching to a lower frequency will generate a wider beam that degrades the lateral resolution.

24. A: Temporal resolution describes the capability of the ultrasound machine to image in real time and is dependent on the frame rate. The frame rate depends on the imaging depth and how many pulses are in each frame. One of the most common steps performed to increase temporal resolution is to decrease the depth during an ultrasound exam. A structure that is located deeper in the body will require a greater time of flight because the system is transmitting the pulses into the body and then back to the transducer to be processed. This additional time will decrease the frame rate and temporal resolution. If the user needs to increase temporal resolution, the scanning depth should always remain as shallow as possible, so there is less time required to process a signal. If a user increases the imaging depth, temporal resolution decreases (slows down) because it takes more time for the signal to return to the system. In other words, an increase in depth decreases the frame rate. When temporal resolution decreases, the operator will notice a lag in the image.

25. D: Refraction is the bending of a sound beam when it travels from one medium to another. Two conditions must apply for refraction to take place in a clinical setting:

1. There must be an oblique angle of incidence
2. The two media must be traveling at different speeds because refraction cannot take place if the media have identical speeds.

Clinically, an ultrasound beam will bend slightly only at various tissue interfaces. Bone tends to create larger refraction angles because the speed of ultrasound in bone is faster than the speed of sound in soft tissues. Snell's law is used to calculate refraction, and the following equation may be used:

$$\frac{\sin(\text{angle of transmission})}{\sin(\text{angle of incidence})} = \frac{\text{speed in medium 2}}{\text{speed in medium 1}}$$

Bernoulli's principle refers to the correlation between velocity and pressure in a fluid. The Curie point refers to the temperature at which polarization of the active element takes place. Huygens' principle explains the hourglass appearance of an ultrasound beam.

26. C: A sonographer can improve the resolution in what appears to be kidney stones (nephrolithiasis) by two methods. If stones are suspected, but distal acoustic shadowing is not clearly identified with a 3 MHz probe, the sonographer can increase the frequency as high as it will go. Higher frequency transducers will create an ultrasound beam that is narrower. If the ultrasound wave is wider than the stone, the beam picks up signals from either side of the stone, and the shadow may not be visualized as well or at all. In this case, perhaps the operator can bump the frequency all the way up to 5 MHz. Another adjustment that can be performed to create a narrow beam is to place the focal point at the depth of the kidney stones. The gain and output power will not affect visualization of the stones.

27. D: The definition of wavelength is the length of one cycle. Wavelength will be displayed in any unit of distance, and the usual range in diagnostic ultrasound imaging is 0.1–0.8 mm. The medium and the sound source are factors that determine the wavelength. Wavelength is not a control on the ultrasound system that a sonographer can change; rather, wavelength changes when changing transducers that have a different frequency. To calculate the wavelength of a sound beam in soft tissue, the following formula can be used:

$$\text{wavelength in soft tissue} = \frac{1.54}{\text{frequency}}.$$

Using this formula, one can visualize the inverse relationship between the wavelength and the frequency, and if the frequency is doubled, the wavelength will be halved, making the only correct choice.

28. B: The backing material is the component of the transducer that will diminish the time (and length) that the PZT crystal is ringing. This layer is attached to the back of the active element to control any excess vibrations. Longer pulses tend to create images with poor axial resolution. Axial resolution will be improved with a shorter pulse length and duration that the crystal is excited. The backing material is also referred to as the damping element and has an impedance that is similar to PZT while retaining much of the energy of the sound (absorption). The matching layer is situated between the patient and the PZT crystal, and it is there to decrease the impedance at the boundary of the skin and the transducer face. The transducer housing is to protect the patient and the user from electrical shock. The wire couples the PZT crystals and the ultrasound machine.

29. C: The purpose of the matching layer is to enable the ultrasound energy to make a smooth transition from the transducer into the patient's body by curbing the reflections at the skin. Ultrasound gel also helps transmit the sound beam into the body by eliminating the air gap. The thickness of the transducer's matching layer should be one-quarter of the wavelength of the sound beam. In this instance, the length of the wavelength is $0.8(1/4) = 0.2$.

30. A: The frequency of sound will travel at the same speed when traveling through the same medium. The speed of sound does not rely on the transducer frequency, only the medium (which is renal tissue in this example). The speed of sound cannot be changed by the operator, so all three frequencies will travel at the same speed if they are within the same tissue. The speed will change only if they are all located in different types of tissues.

31. B: Ultrasound labs use pulsed wave imaging transducers that contain backing material. Backing material (also referred to as damping material) is used to optimize the axial resolution. This is accomplished by attaching a mix of epoxy resin and tungsten particles to the back of the active element or PZT crystal. Using backing material will decrease the sensitivity of the transducer, create a wide bandwidth (range of operating frequencies), and be referred to as having a low quality (Q) factor. The Q-factor refers to the authenticity of the beam. Non-imaging probes do not contain backing material, which creates a narrow bandwidth. Non-imaging probes, for example, CW Doppler and therapeutic ultrasound transducers, are known as having a high Q-factor, which displays a narrow bandwidth.

32. D: The image shape in this question is referred to as a blunted sector. It resembles the classic sector-shaped image at greater depths, but the difference lies at the top of the image. The indentation is associated with the curvature of the transducer face in convex array probes. A linear sequential array produces an image in the shape of a rectangle. A vector array transducer produces an image that is in the shape of a trapezoid. An annular phased array transducer produces images that are sector shaped with a sharp point at the top.

33. B: This image demonstrates an image in which the midportion is lost due to a horizontal band of dropout, which is demonstrated by the black band. The user will still be able to see the rest of the image that is not within this horizontal band. This malfunction has taken place in one of the rings of an annular phased array transducer. If an element malfunctions in either a linear sequential array or a convex sequential array transducer, the result will be a vertical band of dropout beneath the damaged crystal. Recall that a mechanical transducer only has one active element, so if this crystal is damaged, the sonographer will not see an image at all when attempting to scan.

34. C: There are many advantages of using any transducer with phased array technology. Linear phased array probes have small footprints, enabling easier intercostal scanning. Another advantage is that the sonographer can electronically focus the ultrasound beam at all depths during an exam. Focusing can be optimized regardless of the depth of the anatomical structure being interrogated. Steering is also controlled electronically. With linear phased array transducers, the part that touches the patient is flat, but the beam is sent into the body in a nonlinear fashion, creating an image that is sector shaped. In other words, the pulses can also reach structures in the body that are not directly in front of them.

35. A: Annular phased array transducers will have crystals that are shaped like discs, which are arranged in a concentric ring to look like a target. The inner active elements will control focusing at shallower depths. Recall that smaller diameter active elements will produce a beam that is focused at a more superficial region.

Deeper focused beams are produced because crystals with a greater diameter allow this. Each ring in an annular phased array will focus at different depths with each becoming deeper than the one before. The end result is an image that comprises only data from each active element's focal zone. A mechanical transducer does fit the criteria for being steered mechanically, but it will have fixed focusing. Linear sequential and convex sequential array transducers allow electronic multifocusing and electronic steering.

36. D: The Fresnel zone is another name for the near zone or near field of the sound wave. This is the region between the transducer and the focal point (which is where the beam is the narrowest). As the sound wave leaves the transducer, it steadily narrows until it reaches the focus. It is at the focal point where the sound beam is half of the diameter of the crystal. The beam is equal to 13 mm at the transducer face.

37. C: The amount of divergence that occurs in the far field (the Fraunhofer zone) is not determined only by the frequency of the soundwave but also by the diameter of the crystal. The diameter of the crystal and the amount of divergence in the far zone are inversely related. For example, a small crystal diameter results in a beam that generates a greater amount of divergence in the far field. Conversely, a larger diameter PZT crystal will result in a beam that is narrower (a lower amount of divergence). Line density and speed do not affect the amount of divergence. The focal zone depth is directly affected by the frequency and the crystal diameter. For example, if a higher frequency is used, there will be a deeper focal depth. Also, a smaller crystal diameter results in a focal depth that is in a shallower location.

38. B: When using a linear sequential array transducer, the image is rectangular. These modern transducers have the capability of being electronically steered and thus would become shaped like a parallelogram instead of a rectangle. The image will never be wider than the probe's footprint. These transducers have a relatively small footprint, and the PZT crystals are located next to each other across the transducer face. These probes have about 120–250 pieces of the active element used to create the sound beam. Linear phased array and annular phased array transducers generate images that are fan or sector shaped. The convex array produces an image that is known as a blunted sector shape.

39. C: Continuous wave (CW) transducer technology uses two active elements. One crystal is constantly sending out sound waves, whereas the other is always on the receiving end. The location of the signals cannot be determined because everything in the path of the sound wave is being recorded, which means there is a lack of range resolution (also referred to as range ambiguity). These transducers are extremely sensitive in picking up Doppler signals (because they do not have backing material), such as fetal heart tones or ankle pulses, but they cannot be used to generate ultrasound images. The other choices in this question are all examples of imaging transducers that do provide images with range resolution.

40. A: To determine if the beam is steered while using a linear phased array transducer, an imaginary line can be drawn connecting the electrical spikes. A straight line indicates that there is no beam steering. If a rise or fall in the line that connects the electrical spikes is noted, steering of the ultrasound beam has taken place. In this image, a definite slope is apparent as the electrical spikes are moving up when passing from left to right. Next, draw a second imaginary line perpendicular to the slope so a T shape is formed. This demonstrates the direction in which the beam will be steered. In this instance, the beam will be steered 45 degrees to the right. This method can be used even if the beam is focused; however, the electrical spikes will not be in a straight line but will take on a curved appearance.

41. D: Focusing is achieved in linear phased array transducers when the electronic spikes are in a curved configuration, known as the electronic curve. If the electronic spikes are not curved, an unfocused wave is created. The electronic slope determines the direction in which the ultrasound wave will be steered. The dynamic aperture is used in array transducers to change the width of the ultrasound wave. PZT crystals are the active elements that create ringing in the transducer when they are excited.

42. B: Range ambiguity is an imaging error in which returning echoes have not yet been returned to the probe before the next pulse is transmitted. If a sonographer increases the imaging depth, the system automatically decreases the pulse repetition frequency (PRF) to avoid range ambiguity. If the PRF is too high while scanning a structure deep in the body, range ambiguity may occur and the system will incorrectly place the received reflections closer to the probe than their actual depth. PRF represents the number of pulses sent into the body every second and is presented in units of hertz (Hz). The PRF is inversely related to the imaging depth, so if the scan depth is twice as deep, the ultrasound system will automatically reduce the PRF by half. The number of scan lines or the persistence is not affected by the imaging depth. The PRP is also determined by the imaging depth, but they have a direct relationship. For example, if the imaging depth is increased, the PRP will also increase. The PRP is the duration from the beginning of one pulse to the next.

43. A: When a sonographer applies focusing during an exam, many changes take place within the ultrasound beam. Near-zone resolution is enhanced. When focusing is used, the energy of the beam is concentrated into one small area (focus), thus improving the lateral resolution. A focused beam also tends to move the focal point closer to the face of the probe being used. This will result in a near-zone length that is shorter when compared to an unfocused beam. Although the ultrasound beam's shape changes, the width is also changed. The beam's diameter will diverge more in the far field, which diminishes the lateral resolution in the far zone.

44. C: If a sonographer scans a blood vessel with B-mode (also referred to as brightness mode), or grayscale, ultrasound, the image will typically appear anechoic because the reflections are not strong enough for visualization. A structure that is anechoic is free from internal echoes. Of course, the ultrasound operator will use color flow Doppler to provide more information pertaining to the blood flow. Hyperechoic involves structures that appear brighter than neighboring tissues. Isogenic describes tissues that display the same amount of brightness on grayscale imaging. Heterogeneous describes a variance of echoes in the tissue that is being evaluated.

45. B: Ultrasound machines are designed to calculate the speed of the ultrasound wave in soft tissue as 1.54mm/μs. The time of flight (go-return time) refers to the time it takes for a pulse to leave the transducer, hit a reflector, and return to the transducer. The depth of the reflector can be calculated as being 1 cm when the time of flight equals 13 μs. Using this rule, if a target is 2 cm deep, the time of flight will be twice as long, equating to 26 μs. If the time of flight takes 39μs, the depth of the reflector will be 3 cm.

46. D: Grayscale imaging requires the use of pulsed wave ultrasound to create an image. Recall that continuous wave (CW) ultrasound, although extremely sensitive, cannot produce an image. Clinically, pulsed wave ultrasound enables the ultrasound system to determine the depth of the reflector by calculating the go-return time, which enables image production. A shorter go-return time correlates with a reflector that is at a shallower depth than one that has a longer go-return time, which is associated with a reflector that is located deeper in the body. Penetration is determined by the output power. Temporal resolution is affected by the imaging depth because a greater depth will result in poorer temporal resolution. The bandwidth refers to the available frequencies in the pulse.

47. C: When the user adjusts the receiver gain on an ultrasound system, it is the amplification that is modified. This action takes place in the receiver, and it has a uniform effect on the image by changing the strength of the voltages that the probe has produced. If the receiver gain is increased, a brighter image will appear throughout the entire image. If the gain is decreased, the overall image becomes darker. Demodulation cannot be adjusted by the user. Reject discards the weak signals. Compression is used to modify the grayscale maps.

48. C: M-mode (also referred to as motion mode) is commonly used during echocardiograms to evaluate heart valve and wall motion as the heart is beating. It is also used to obtain a fetal heart rate during obstetrical ultrasounds. The information that is depicted during M-mode is the amplitude, motion, and time. The user will witness lines moving across the screen when M-mode is employed. Time is represented by the *x*-axis. The *y*-axis correlates with the depth of the reflector, and the brightness of the dots corresponds to the amplitude. M-mode displays excellent temporal resolution because only one line is being assessed. Depth and amplitude describe A-mode (also referred to as amplitude mode) with the *x*-axis representing the depth and the *y*-axis corresponding to the amplitude. B-mode is grayscale imaging with the depth being determined by the *x*-axis and amplitude correlating to the *z*-axis.

49. B: The dynamic range is a ratio of signals that can be portrayed by a system while still containing accurate information. This controls how the intensity of the signals is transformed into shades of gray. This will either increase or limit the different shades of gray. If the image displayed on an ultrasound system has a high amount of contrast, it means that the pixels are either black or white. High-contrast images portray few shades of gray. Therefore, if only black and white are displayed, then there is a narrow dynamic range. A dynamic range that shows many shades of gray would be considered to have a wide dynamic range. These images will be considered to be of low contrast.

50. D: Output gain is one of several names that describes the power of the ultrasound system. Other names for power include output power, output, and acoustic power. The pulser is the component of the ultrasound system that regulates the intensity of the beam that the patient is exposed to. A higher output gain (power) will also increase the ability to scan at greater depths while decreasing the amount of noise present during the scan. Pulse duration and frequency are not related to the output gain used during the exam.

51. A: Tissue harmonics is a technology that is available to correct the malformation of the ultrasound wave that takes place as the sound wave travels into the body. The transmitted, or fundamental, frequency is the frequency of the ultrasound beam that is produced by the transducer and imparted into the patient, and it is responsible for image production. However, during tissue harmonics, this frequency tends to be excluded so that the only signal being used is the harmonic frequency. The harmonic frequency is created within the patient's body and will be two times larger than the fundamental frequency, improving contrast resolution. For example, if the fundamental frequency is 6 MHz, the harmonic frequency will be 12 MHz. An ultrasound beam that is created with harmonic frequencies will not undergo as much distortion and is less likely to produce images with artifacts. When harmonics are used, a strong signal is required, and these signals will be located within the main axis of the sound wave. Spatial compounding can be used to eliminate edge shadows. Overall gain is another name for the process of amplification.

52. B: The gallbladder is an organ that is subject to image artifacts when scanned with ultrasound. It can be difficult to discern if reflectors visualized within it are real. Tissue harmonics is a concept that has helped clinicians and operators gain diagnostic confidence because it tends to eliminate some signals that are not pathological. Harmonic frequencies allow the sonographer to scan patients at higher frequencies that will not only improve the axial resolution but the lateral resolution as well. The lateral resolution tends to improve because the wave is narrower. The use of harmonic frequencies makes it easier to image gallbladders and those organs that are deeper in the body, and it eliminates reverberation artifacts. Reverberation artifacts can mimic sludge within the gallbladder.

53. C: Write zoom can also be referred to as write magnification. This is a type of zoom that can be performed before the image is stored in the scan converter, which makes this a preprocessing function. The spatial resolution is superior because once the image is converted from analog to digital, only the information within the region of interest will be scanned again, creating more pixels and thus resulting in better spatial resolution. Read magnification is a postprocessing function because it can be performed only on an image that has been frozen. This results in pixels that are bigger than the original and will not improve the resolution. Read magnification is also known as read zoom. Temporal resolution can be referred to as the frame rate and may be better if write magnification is used.

54. A: If a sonographer notices that the image is being affected by electronic noise, it may be necessary to adjust the reject on the ultrasound system. The reject function is also referred to as rejection, threshold, or even suppression. Reject is the last process that takes place in the receiver. This function is typically offered in two forms: one that takes place automatically and one that can be controlled by the operator. The reject enables the user to decide if low-level echoes should be displayed within the image, but it does not suppress brighter signals. Sometimes, weaker signals will offer important data for a diagnosis, but clinicians often do not want noise to be present on the image. When the sonographer adjusts the amplification, the whole image will become brighter or darker. Compression allows the user to select the grayscale maps. Demodulation cannot be controlled by the sonographer, and it does not affect the appearance of the ultrasound exam.

55. D: If a sonographer finds it necessary to improve an image while scanning the kidneys (renal ultrasound), it is possible for the operator to adjust the output power, which controls the intensity of the beam. The amplitude can also be modified by increasing or decreasing the amount of receiver gain. The frequency can also be adjusted by increasing or decreasing the frequency that a particular transducer offers or by switching probes. The speed of sound does not depend on any component of the ultrasound machine, but rather the medium, and it cannot be changed by the sonographer. The speed will change only if the type of tissue changes.

56. C: An application that can be used to assist in better visualization of fibroids is coded excitation, which occurs in the pulser. Penetration and resolution are two important factors when considering the quality of an ultrasound image. Higher resolution is obtained using short pulses during an ultrasound exam. Coded excitation allows longer pulses across a variety of frequencies to improve the resolution and allow for deeper penetration, which is often necessary when scanning uterine fibroids. It is possible to apply multiple focal zones with coded excitation. With better penetration and increased resolution in the far field, fibroids are easier to correctly diagnose when using transvaginal transducers. Persistence uses data from images that have already been acquired to improve the quality of the image. Spatial compounding generates an image by acquiring data from angles that can eliminate certain artifacts and can be performed only with phased array technology. Elastography provides information pertaining to the stiffness of the structure being examined.

57. B: If the sharpness of a subtle mass located within the liver needs to be improved, edge enhancement can be applied. This is a technique that allows for better delineation of the border of structures by sharpening the edges of a mass. Edge enhancement sharpens the borders by raising the amount of image contrast at the interface of these tissues. At the boundary between two or more tissue types, shades of gray are displayed, and edge enhancement portrays edges that are more reflective to help the mass stand out more against normal liver tissue that can be identified in the background. Zoom is a technique that is used to magnify an image or part of an image. Fill-in interpolation is a preprocessing technique that provides information about missing data based on what is located between scan lines. If the sonographer increases the receiver gain, this will make the entire image brighter.

58. D: This ultrasound beam has been created with a linear phased array transducer, which is focused and steered to the left. When examining the picture, it is important to note that there is a curvature of the electrical spikes. This curved design governs the focusing of a phased array transducer, which is present. If it were an unfocused beam, the electrical spikes would be in a straight line. Next, it is necessary to determine the direction in which the beam is being steered, which can be done by drawing a straight line and connecting the spikes from left to right. Intersect this line with another that is perpendicular (90 degrees) to discern the direction in which the beam will be steered (in this case, to the left).

59. C: Frequency compounding is an averaging method that tends to take the speckle patterns of multiple images into consideration to reduce the noise and speckle that are produced. Ultrasound images are filled with speckle, but it is important that a reduction takes place to discern objects that demonstrate low contrast. Targets that are smaller may not be visualized if the amount of speckle is not reduced. Spatial compounding can reduce the amount of shadowing and speckle, but instead of averaging multiple frequencies, this method includes data from various angles. Tissue harmonics develop within the patient and are generated within the main ultrasound beam. Temporal compounding is also known as persistence, and although it can be useful to reduce the speckle pattern, it overlaps data from prior frame rates onto the most recent information to smooth out the image.

60. D: The receiver is one of the main components of the ultrasound machine. The receiver is responsible for changing and displaying the signal that is sent from the transducer to the monitor or whichever type of viewing format is being used. This is the fourth component after the transducer, pulser, and beam former, which, as the name suggests, shapes the ultrasound beam. The master synchronizer controls the collaboration of the synergy of the ultrasound components, and storage is the component that is responsible for saving the images and video clips.

61. A: The receiver (also known as the signal processor) has five functions that occur during image production. The receiver obtains the echoes after they have been sent into the patient but before this information is sent to the monitor. Note that these functions are in alphabetical order to help recall them, which puts the

129

series in the following order: amplification, compensation, compression, demodulation, and reject. It should be noted that the modification of the receiver operations does not affect patient exposure because these steps take place when the signal is leaving the patient. Of these functions, demodulation is the only one that cannot be modified with a control on the machine and has no effect on the appearance of the image.

62. B: Preprocessing should be thought of as any change of the image that occurs before the user freezes the image. Examples of preprocessing are adjusting the TGC or gain. Preprocessing occurs before the data are sent to the scan converter to be stored. The scan converter is responsible for taking a number and converting the information to grayscale. The pulser determines the intensity of the ultrasound beam. The receiver receives the signal from the patient and prepares it for image display. The beam former works with phased array transducers and determines how the ultrasound beam will be steered and focused.

63. C: Persistence (also called temporal averaging or temporal compounding) is a method that can be used during grayscale or color Doppler imaging. It can be adjusted by the user. By overlapping information obtained from older frames onto more recent images obtained, the machine can produce an ultrasound image with greater detail that has less noise, is smoother, and has an improved signal-to-noise ratio. If the signal-to-noise ratio is higher than the useless low-level echoes, the system will get rid of the noise. Less noise is desired during image production. Although the image detail improves with the use of temporal compounding, temporal resolution is degraded because of the additional processing. This makes imaging structures that are moving rapidly difficult to image because there will be a lag as temporal resolution is decreased. Persistence is best used with structures that demonstrate slow motion, such as slow blood flow.

64. B: Voxel stands for volume element, and it is the smallest element of a picture that has been generated with 3D technology. The difference between a voxel and a pixel is that the latter refers to a 2D image. Pixels are the tiny boxes that will each have their own gray shade to make up a digital image. To produce an image with greater resolution, a higher pixel density is required. Pixel density is the number of boxes per inch on the display. A high pixel density will offer better resolution because there will be more pixels found in every inch of the image. A bit has a value equal to either 1 or 0, and it refers to the smallest unit of data that a computer can store. Bit is the abbreviation for binary digit. In computer language, there are 8 bits in 1 byte.

65. D: The Digital Imaging and Communications in Medicine (DICOM) system is the necessary link between the ultrasound machine (or any other digital imaging system) and the picture archiving and communications system (PACS), the component responsible for archiving and transferring images. DICOM allows for the integration of a facility's networks, printing devices, workstations, and PACS system. The DICOM protocols allow the ultrasound machine to send the images to the PACS network for archiving purposes. In contrast to JPEG images, DICOM images are extremely large, and they cannot be loaded onto regular computers. A DICOM browser is necessary so that the images can be viewed on computers, workstations, or even a CD. A bit is the smallest unit of information in computer language. RIS is an acronym for radiology information system, which is an electronic health record specific to radiology departments for scheduling, tracking patients, and billing functions.

66. B: PACS allows users of digital imaging equipment to electronically share and archive images. This is an important tool that gives clinicians and other medical personnel access to images as well reports that have been generated. PACS has been used to replace film for facilities that have converted to digital imaging systems. This not only saves storage space for film and chemicals used to process film within departments, but it also allows more than one user to visualize studies at the same time as well as it grants instantaneous access to the stored images. Over time, film studies tend to deteriorate; this will not occur with studies that are archived with a PACS system. RIS is an electronic health record specific to radiology departments for scheduling, tracking patients, and billing functions. A bit is the smallest unit of information in computer language. DICOM is a necessary link between the ultrasound machine (or any other digital imaging system) and the PACS system, and it allows for the integration of the facility's networks, printing devices, workstations, and PACS system.

67. D: The progression of the signal through an ultrasound machine is first the transducer, which contains the PZT crystal. Next is the receiver, which will change the probe's electrical signal so that it can eventually be visualized on the monitor. The scan converter is responsible for changing the data from analog to digital, and digital to analog, as well as controlling the system's memory. The display is the component that allows the operator to view the images generated by the system.

68. A: A pixel is the smallest portion of a 2D image that is in a digital format. Pixel density refers to the number of pixels contained in every inch of the image. The more pixels that an image contains, the better the spatial resolution. A high pixel density will dramatically improve an image, whether it is on a digital camera, flat-screen TV, or ultrasound display. In this example, analog and digital display are added as additional information to throw the reader off, but if better spatial resolution is desired, the user must choose the 1,500 × 1,500 analog display because of the higher pixel count that generates 2,250,000 pixels (multiply 1,500 × 1,500).

69. C: If the radiologist requests an image with as much anatomy as possible, the sonographer could use the extended field of view (EFOV) control on the ultrasound system. This application can be used when interrogating a Baker's cyst, the length of the Achilles tendon, or the abdominal aorta to provide additional information regarding the exact location of aneurysms or other pathology that may be encountered. This panoramic image is available on most modern ultrasound equipment and replaces the split-screen method of demonstrating objects that are longer than the transducer face. By acquiring volume data, the system will stitch the information together to display one image. Often, anatomical structures are enlarged, and it may be difficult to obtain measurements. Other uses include exams of the thyroid, testes, or breast lesions, and musculoskeletal exams, . Elastography is an application that measures tissue stiffness. Color Doppler will typically be used during evaluation of the abdominal aorta, but this application provides information related to the Doppler shift of the blood flow. B-mode is grayscale imaging, which is used to generate ultrasound images, but EFOV is the choice that will allow the greatest field of view.

70. A: The horizontal axis of a TGC curve refers to how much compensation is necessary for the depth of the object being imaged (vertical axis). The top of the vertical axis represents the patient's skin, and as it moves down, it refers to tissues that are located deeper in the body. The near gain is located superficially near the skin's surface. At this location, the structures being imaged need little TGC because not much attenuation occurs. The slope is the middle portion of the TGC curve in which more compensation is necessary because of the greater depths. The knee is located at the distal portion of the slope, and it demonstrates where the most compensation will occur. The region of the far gain is distal to the knee and even deeper, which designates the greatest amount of compensation offered by the machine. Phase quadrature is not a component of the TGC curve.

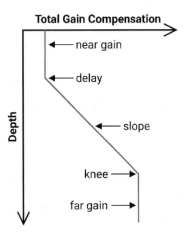

71. B: A bit has a value equal to either 1 or 0, and it is the smallest unit of data that a computer can store. To calculate the number of shades of gray in 3 bits of memory, one would take 2 to the nth power, with n equal to the number of bits. In this instance, $2^3 = 2 \times 2 \times 2 = 8$. This demonstrates that in 3 bits of memory, one can see eight different shades of gray.

72. D: Contrast resolution can be thought of as the ability to see the differences in intensities in tissues that are beside each other on a grayscale image. Ultrasound images that contain many shades of gray will offer better contrast resolution. To calculate the number of shades of gray in a specific number of bits of memory, one would take 2 to the nth power, with n equal to the number of bits. Four bits is equal to 2 to the 4th power ($2 \times 2 \times 2 \times 2$), which is equal to 16 different shades of gray. Two hundred fifty-six shades of gray would be 2 to the 8th power, which is equal to

8 bits. Thirty-two shades of gray would be 2 to the 5th power, which is 5 bits. Sixteen bits is equal to 65,536 shades of gray, so, of the options listed, this will offer the highest amount of gray shades and provide the best contrast resolution.

73. D: During a carotid duplex exam, if a sonographer is using pulsed wave Doppler to determine the peak velocity of blood flow in a carotid artery, the operator must remember that when the red blood cells are moving along the same path of the ultrasound beam, the most accurate measurements will be obtained. Thus, the Doppler shift (otherwise known as the Doppler frequency) will be highest at 0 (flow moving toward the transducer) or 180 degrees (flow moving away from the transducer). If the angle between the target and reflector is anything other than 0 or 180 degrees, the velocity is less precise. If an operator tries to interrogate a structure at a 90-degree angle with pulsed wave Doppler, no Doppler shift will take place because the frequency shift cannot be identified because the cosine of 90 degrees is equal to 0.

74. C: When an ultrasound operator wants to measure velocities within a blood vessel, pulsed wave Doppler can be used. The advantage of pulsed wave (over CW) Doppler is that the sonographer can place the gate (sample volume) in a location of choice to obtain the best measurements. The gate should be placed in the center of the blood vessel.

75. C: This is a spectral Doppler waveform of the patient's left internal carotid artery (ICA) that indicates a significant amount of plaque in the proximal portion of the left ICA. This spectral waveform of the mid-left ICA displays a peak systolic velocity (PSV) of 479.6 cm/s, with an end-diastolic velocity (EDV) of 151.7 cm/s. Because the PSV is greater than 125 cm/s and the EDV is more than 140 cm/s, it is estimated that the diameter reduction of the left ICA is 80–99%. The Doppler signal was obtained with the angle correction of 60 degrees, and the sample volume was placed distal to the stenosis. The waveform also demonstrates a considerable amount of spectral broadening.

76. B: The pressure within the venous system is influenced by a patient's breathing patterns due to the fact that it is a low-pressure system and due to the movement of the diaphragm with inspiration and expiration. If a sonographer asks the patient to take in a deep breath and hold it, this is referred to as inhalation, or inspiration. With inspiration, venous flow rate in the legs decreases because the diaphragm descends into the abdominal cavity. This downward movement of the diaphragm increases pressure within the abdominal cavity. Conversely, upon expiration, the diaphragm ascends into the chest cavity, which decreases venous blood flow from above the level of the heart while increasing the amount of pressure in the chest. Turbulent flow is often present distal to a stenosis. Pulsatile flow is associated with the contraction of the heart and is typically present when evaluating the arterial system with Doppler.

77. A: Sonographers should immediately identify these images as typical blood flow patterns in which the red blood cells are moving through the vessel when no pathology is present. Laminar flow is the type of flow that is exhibited in normal anatomical structures. This flow is layered and smooth and travels parallel along the length of the vessel. There are two configurations regarding laminar flow. The first picture represents a parabolic pattern that tends to have velocities that are higher in the middle of the vessel with slower velocity flow along the walls. The shape that is created with a parabolic flow pattern is like a bullet. The second image demonstrates plug flow, which will have the same velocity in all of the layers present. A blood vessel that contains laminar flow will produce a Reynolds number of less than 1,500. The Reynolds number is a way to forecast if the flow will be laminar or turbulent. Turbulent flow will have a Reynolds number that is greater than 2,000. Turbulent flow is also associated with chaotic blood flow and eddy currents.

78. A: The 14 MHz transducer will display a Doppler shift that is greater than that of the 7 MHz transducer. Higher frequency transducers generate greater Doppler shifts, and there is a direct relationship between the Doppler shift and transducer frequency. In this instance, the Doppler shift was doubled when switching from a 7 MHz to a 14 MHz transducer. If the sonographer would have started with a 14 MHz transducer and then used the 7 MHz probe, the Doppler shift would have been halved.

79. C: The error that is depicted in this image is known as aliasing. Aliasing is a common artifact witnessed in color Doppler and in spectral Doppler. There are many steps that can be taken to eliminate signals that display aliasing. The first step a sonographer should try is to adjust the pulse repetition frequency (PRF), which is also known as the velocity scale. Because this is an artery, the blood flow is moving rapidly, so increasing the PRF may help unwrap the spectral display. This step increases the Nyquist limit, which is also known as the aliasing frequency and is equal to half of the PRF. If this alone does not take care of aliasing, the baseline may be adjusted accordingly. In this situation, dropping the baseline down closer to the bottom of the window will help alleviate the appearance of aliasing. Another helpful tip to eliminate aliasing is to switch to a lower frequency transducer or even to find a window that is at a shallower location. The sonographer could also use continuous wave (CW) Doppler because aliasing will never occur, since aliasing is exclusively inherent with pulsed Doppler.

80. A: Pulsed wave Doppler is a useful method to measure blood flow velocities within blood vessels. The user has the option to select where the gate should be placed within a vessel to take a velocity measurement and know the exact location of this reading. However, sometimes the velocity within the blood vessel is too high, and the operator is unable to obtain a peak velocity measurement that is accurate. The sonographer would want to switch to continuous wave (CW) Doppler because velocities that are extremely high tend to be more accurate because there will not be a maximum velocity while using this method. While using pulsed wave Doppler, if the user cannot eliminate aliasing after changing the scale or depth of the target or switching to a lower frequency probe, one will be successful if switching to CW Doppler.

81. D: The aliasing frequency is also referred to as the Nyquist limit. This number can be calculated by dividing the pulse repetition frequency (PRF) by 2. Aliasing will be apparent if the Doppler frequency is higher than the Nyquist limit. Therefore, to prevent aliasing, the sonographer will want to raise the Nyquist limit. This can be done by raising the PRF scale: If the PRF is increased, so is the Nyquist limit. One may also raise the Nyquist limit by finding a new sonographic window that is at a shallower location. The PRF is controlled by the reflector depth. If the target is deeper in the body, the PRF will be low, as will the Nyquist limit. This decreased value makes the ultrasound system more susceptible to aliasing. When we divide the PRF (which is 8) by 2, it equals 4 kHz.

82. C: Color Doppler is a pulsed wave technique that demonstrates a Doppler frequency shift that overlays a grayscale image with the use of autocorrelation. Color Doppler is a pulsed wave technique; therefore, aliasing may occur. Due to it being a pulsed wave method, range resolution does exist when using color Doppler. Color Doppler is not used to measure the peak systolic and end diastolic velocities but rather the mean velocity and direction of a moving target.

83. B: PRF stands for pulse repetition frequency but is also referred to as the scale while pulsed Doppler is being used. In this example, the vessel being interrogated displays blood flow that is moving slowly. If color is not optimized after turning on color Doppler, the sonographer would want to decrease the PRF so that the ultrasound system is more receptive in picking up slower blood flow signals. Blood that is within the venous portion of the circulatory system is often blood that moves more slowly. If this step alone does not improve the color Doppler visualization of the vessel, the sonographer may need to increase the color gain. If the operator chose to increase the PRF scale, a decreased sensitivity to slow flow will be noted. However, if one is interrogating a vessel with higher velocity flow, the PRF should be set higher to raise the Nyquist limit and prevent or eliminate aliasing. Adjusting the PRF does affect the visualization of blood flow, which makes incorrect.

84. A: In general, a Doppler shift is produced when an ultrasound wave collides with a red blood cell that is in motion, which means that a Doppler shift is absolutely present. It must be determined, however, if the shift will be positive or negative. If the red blood cells are traveling in a direction that is in the opposite direction of the transducer, a negative Doppler shift would take place. When the red blood cells are moving in the direction of the transducer, the result is a frequency that is reflected and is greater than the frequency of the transmitted signal. This demonstrates a positive Doppler shift (also known as the Doppler frequency). The amount of Doppler shift that occurs is directly proportional to the frequency of the transducer. Therefore, if an exam is repeated with a transducer that has a frequency that is twice as high as what was used in the first exam, the Doppler shift (frequency) will be doubled. Unequivocal is not a viable option for this question.

85. C: Aliasing occurs when the spectral waveform tends to wind around the spectral window. Carotid duplex exams are performed with linear sequential transducers. Aliasing will be eliminated when a lower frequency transducer is being used, and, in this example, if the sonographer started with 10 MHz, the next step would be to switch to the 7 MHz linear sequential transducer. A 4.5 MHz curved array transducer, although a lower frequency, is not a transducer that is used to complete carotid exams. Higher frequency probes are more prone to aliasing artifacts because the Doppler shift is calculated using the frequency of the transducer and, in turn, it has a direct relationship. Doppler shifts will be smaller when lower frequency probes are used, so aliasing does not occur as often with lower frequency transducers.

86. B: When a sonographer is using routine grayscale ultrasound imaging, it has been proven that the ideal incident beam is when the transducer is placed 90 degrees to the object being scanned. By using the Doppler equation, however, the cosine of 90 degrees is equal to 0. This indicates that the ultrasound system will not pick up a Doppler frequency when the angle of incidence is 90 degrees (perpendicular) to the direction of blood flow and needs to be changed. If the sonographer saw the movement of blood cells on grayscale imaging, this is a great clue that the blood vessel is not obstructed. Although using power Doppler is an option, it is important to try to optimize color Doppler first because power Doppler does not provide information pertaining to the direction or speed of blood flow. Calling maintenance is likely not necessary unless several attempts of modifying the angle of incidence, increasing the color gain, and adjusting the scale fail to demonstrate color. If this is still the case, one may conclude that the color Doppler is not working correctly and maintenance should be called.

87. A: If a sonographer notices that the lower velocities are missing from the spectral waveform, the wall filter control can be decreased so that the lower frequency shifts appear along the baseline. It is important to note that the wall filter does not affect blood flow that is moving at a higher velocity and tends to get rid of the shifts that are the result of anatomical motion. The scale is the pulse repetition frequency (PRF), and this can be adjusted if the spectral waveform is aliasing. If aliasing occurs, the scale should be increased. Changing the depth will not help demonstrate the lower frequency velocities. The gain of the spectral Doppler waveform can be increased or decreased, but this will affect only the appearance of the grayscale data within the spectral window and is used to eliminate any noise that may be evident.

88. D: The Reynolds number is a value that predicts the flow patterns of blood; it is a unitless number that be calculated from the following equation:

$$\text{Reynolds number} = \frac{(\text{average flow speed}) \times (\text{vessel diameter}) \times (\text{density})}{(\text{viscosity})}$$

If the calculated value is less than 1,500, laminar flow will be present. It should be noted that plug flow is a type of laminar flow. Disturbed flow will fall between 1,500 and 2,000. If the value is more than 2,000 it is predicted that turbulent flow will be visualized, and in this instance, the flow is predicted to be turbulent because it is 2,078. As seen with the equation, if there is increased speed of flow, there will be a higher Reynolds number. If the diameter of the vessel is larger, the Reynolds number will also be greater. Density has the same effect on this calculation. The Reynolds number has an indirect relationship with the viscosity of the blood.

89. C: During a carotid duplex exam, if color appears to be bleeding outside of the artery when color Doppler is applied, it is known as a ghosting artifact. Ghosting and clutter are both low-frequency Doppler shifts that initiate artifacts from anatomical motion, such as the arterial wall. Clutter is associated with the spectral waveform, and when this low-frequency shift is seen with color Doppler, it is referred to as ghosting. Crosstalk is seen on a spectral display only when blood flow appears bidirectional when it truly is unidirectional. Pulsed Doppler can create aliasing, which is the most prevalent artifact when color or spectral Doppler is used.

90. A: Spectral analysis with pulsed wave Doppler allows users to see, hear, and measure blood flow velocities. The spectral window is the clear, black region between the baseline and the spectral line. When this area is filled in and there is widening of the line, spectral broadening is indicated. Spectral broadening is typical when turbulent (high-velocity) blood flow is sampled. This turbulence comprises many areas of flow reversal and velocities, and flow may be seen beneath the baseline. If the ICA is being interrogated and the sonographer can visualize a tight stenosis, one would not be surprised to see spectral broadening. Instead of a clear spectral window, which is expected in a patent ICA or laminar flow, it appears to be filled in, which represents spectral broadening. If the gain is set too high, noise will be apparent throughout the entire window.

91. B: Sometimes, the sonographer will notice that blood flow from arteries and veins is being displayed. Modern systems will have a triplex function that allows the user to display grayscale, color Doppler, and spectral Doppler at the same time. If the user is picking up flow from two different vessels, they should update the triplex image, and move the sample volume into the vessel of interest. Angle correction is necessary to measure the velocities of the blood within a vessel. The sweep speed controls the number of seconds that are shown at once. Pulse repetition frequency (PRF) is the scale that represents the pulses generated every second by the system.

92. D: Color Doppler will allow velocity information to be portrayed as an overlay of color on the traditional grayscale image. To optimize temporal resolution, the user needs to be aware of the size and location of the color box. As the color box size increases, the frame rate, or temporal resolution, decreases because more information needs to be processed. This is especially important when considering the width of the color box. More scan lines are required with a wider color box, and more time is required by the system to process the acquired data. The sonographer should limit the size of the color box to the anatomy of interest and most importantly decrease the width of the color box. The location is also something to consider because a deeper location may be prone to aliasing of the color flow because the pulse repetition frequency (PRF) is lower. The angle of the color box and gain will not affect temporal resolution.

93. B: During a Doppler exam, the only choice that will increase the amount of exposure for the patient in this instance is if the sonographer increases the pulse repetition frequency (PRF). PRF is a control that sonographers are familiar with when using color and pulsed wave Doppler imaging. PRF controls how rapidly data sampling takes place and will allow the ultrasound system to increase or decrease the Doppler shifts that are displayed. A high PRF setting enables more sampling to take place because there is less listening time between the pulses, which equates to more pulses transmitted into the body. It is important to have the PRF set correctly during both modalities so that aliasing does not occur. Color Doppler enables ultrasound users to determine the direction of flow when present and requires eight pulses/scan line. Spectral analysis allows operators to measure velocities as well as provides information about the direction and presence of flow but requires more effort at 256 pulses/scan line. Increasing the Doppler angle, repositioning the baseline to a higher location, and increasing the Doppler gain will not affect the amount of exposure to the patient.

94. C: Pulse repetition frequency (PRF) is the number of pulses sent in one second. When color Doppler is used, many pulses are used for each scan line to increase the sensitivity to low flow and to get a more precise measurement of the velocities. In this instance, the sonographer would want to decrease the packet size to improve the frame rate because less time is required with a smaller packet size. The packet size is also referred to as the ensemble length. An increased packet size tends to degrade temporal resolution because more pulses are being sent out at the same time, which requires more time for data acquisition. Changing the color map and adjusting the color Doppler gain will not affect the frame rate.

95. A: Power Doppler (also referred to as energy mode or color angio) is a form of color Doppler that does not display the speed of blood flow or any directional information. Hence, power Doppler does not evaluate the velocity of the blood flow. Rather, it determines only that a Doppler shift has taken place and shows the amplitude of the moving blood. If there are more red blood cells in one area, the signals will be brighter. Vessels represented with power Doppler will all be identical colors on the display. Advantages of power Doppler include the fact that aliasing does not occur because the speed and direction (velocity) of the blood flow are not applicable. Power Doppler picks up blood flow in smaller vessels and slow blood flow because of its increase in sensitivity. There is an increase in sensitivity because power Doppler is not altered by the Doppler angle.

96. D: Ultrasound operators have several options to eliminate signals that display aliasing. The first step a sonographer should try is to adjust the pulse repetition frequency (PRF,). In this instance, blood is moving through the femoral artery rapidly, so increasing the PRF may help to unwrap the spectral display. This step increases the Nyquist limit, which is also known as the aliasing frequency and is equal to half of the PRF. If this alone does not take care of aliasing, the baseline may be adjusted accordingly. Another helpful tip to eliminate aliasing is to switch to a lower frequency transducer or even find a window that is at a shallower location. The angle of incidence could also be increased to help eliminate aliasing.

97. B: Aliasing can occur with not only spectral Doppler analysis but with color flow Doppler as well. Sonographers must be able to discern between aliasing and the reversal of flow (bidirectional flow). To determine if aliasing is present in the carotid artery, the user must pay close attention to the color map located on the side of the image. If the colors on the map tend to wrap from the top around the outside and to the bottom of the map, then users may assume that aliasing is present. If the colors on the middle of the color map communicate with each other, as stated in this example, then bidirectional flow is present. The wall filter affects only slow flow, which would not affect the blood moving within the carotid artery.

98. B: Color Doppler in a sector-shaped image cannot be steered like it can with a linear transducer. Only the size and location of the color box can be adjusted. Steering of the color box in this instance cannot be performed as it could if a linear transducer were in use. The shape of the color box cannot be changed as it may with a linear transducer when it changes from a rectangle to a parallelogram when steering is employed. The velocities of the moving red blood cells can be determined.

99. A: In this image, note that the color box is almost perpendicular to the blood vessel (but it is not quite 90 degrees, which is why some flow is visible within the lumen while not being completely filled in). The cosine of 90 degrees is equal to 0, which means that no Doppler shift can be detected. Color Doppler works best when the angle between the ultrasound beam and the blood flow is something other than 90 degrees and will enable the machine to display color flow in the blood vessels that are being interrogated. One of the first steps that a sonographer would take in this instance is to change the steering of the color box. It is already steered to the right, but the direction should be changed, and because the vessel is slanted, it should be steered to the left. Another check that a sonographer can do after adjusting the steering is to increase the color gain, which is the opposite of what states. Increasing the output power will not help the color fill of this vessel. Sometimes finding a window that is shallower will help color Doppler, but it is not typically the first step to improve flow.

100. C: Spectral analysis with pulsed wave Doppler allows users to see, hear, and measure blood flow velocities. The spectral window is the clear, black region between the baseline and the spectral line. When this area is filled in and there is widening of the line, spectral broadening is indicated. Spectral broadening is typical when turbulent (high-velocity) blood flow is sampled. This turbulence comprises many areas of flow reversal and velocities, and flow may be seen beneath the baseline. If a velocity measurement is taken within a tight stenosis of the ICA, one would not be surprised to see spectral broadening. This may also be present when small vessels are being investigated or if a velocity is measured distal to a tight stenosis of the ECA. If a sample is obtained in which a vessel bifurcates, it would not be surprising to see spectral broadening. A patent blood vessel is one that is not obstructed, and this is not an instance of when the ultrasound operator would expect to see spectral broadening.

Image Credits

LICENSED UNDER CC BY 4.0 (CREATIVECOMMONS.ORG/LICENSES/BY/4.0/)

Extended Field of View: "panoramic view of an obstructive FLUTD" by Wikimedia user Kalumet
(https://commons.wikimedia.org/wiki/File:FLUTD_Sono_Panoramic_view.jpg)

LICENSED UNDER CC BY-SA 3.0 (CREATIVECOMMONS.ORG/LICENSES/BY-SA/3.0/)

Gallstones: "Gallstones" by James Heilman, MD
(https://commons.wikimedia.org/wiki/File:Gallstones.PNG)

Stenosis: "Internal carotid artery stenosis" by Wikimedia user Mme Mim
(https://commons.wikimedia.org/wiki/File:Internal_carotid_artery_stenosis_in_ultrasound_near_occlusion.jpg)

How to Overcome Test Anxiety

Just the thought of taking a test is enough to make most people a little nervous. A test is an important event that can have a long-term impact on your future, so it's important to take it seriously and it's natural to feel anxious about performing well. But just because anxiety is normal, that doesn't mean that it's helpful in test taking, or that you should simply accept it as part of your life. Anxiety can have a variety of effects. These effects can be mild, like making you feel slightly nervous, or severe, like blocking your ability to focus or remember even a simple detail.

If you experience test anxiety—whether severe or mild—it's important to know how to beat it. To discover this, first you need to understand what causes test anxiety.

Causes of Test Anxiety

While we often think of anxiety as an uncontrollable emotional state, it can actually be caused by simple, practical things. One of the most common causes of test anxiety is that a person does not feel adequately prepared for their test. This feeling can be the result of many different issues such as poor study habits or lack of organization, but the most common culprit is time management. Starting to study too late, failing to organize your study time to cover all of the material, or being distracted while you study will mean that you're not well prepared for the test. This may lead to cramming the night before, which will cause you to be physically and mentally exhausted for the test. Poor time management also contributes to feelings of stress, fear, and hopelessness as you realize you are not well prepared but don't know what to do about it.

Other times, test anxiety is not related to your preparation for the test but comes from unresolved fear. This may be a past failure on a test, or poor performance on tests in general. It may come from comparing yourself to others who seem to be performing better or from the stress of living up to expectations. Anxiety may be driven by fears of the future—how failure on this test would affect your educational and career goals. These fears are often completely irrational, but they can still negatively impact your test performance.

> **Review Video: 3 Reasons You Have Test Anxiety**
> Visit mometrix.com/academy and enter code: 428468

142

Elements of Test Anxiety

As mentioned earlier, test anxiety is considered to be an emotional state, but it has physical and mental components as well. Sometimes you may not even realize that you are suffering from test anxiety until you notice the physical symptoms. These can include trembling hands, rapid heartbeat, sweating, nausea, and tense muscles. Extreme anxiety may lead to fainting or vomiting. Obviously, any of these symptoms can have a negative impact on testing. It is important to recognize them as soon as they begin to occur so that you can address the problem before it damages your performance.

> **Review Video: 3 Ways to Tell You Have Test Anxiety**
> Visit mometrix.com/academy and enter code: 927847

The mental components of test anxiety include trouble focusing and inability to remember learned information. During a test, your mind is on high alert, which can help you recall information and stay focused for an extended period of time. However, anxiety interferes with your mind's natural processes, causing you to blank out, even on the questions you know well. The strain of testing during anxiety makes it difficult to stay focused, especially on a test that may take several hours. Extreme anxiety can take a huge mental toll, making it difficult not only to recall test information but even to understand the test questions or pull your thoughts together.

> **Review Video: How Test Anxiety Affects Memory**
> Visit mometrix.com/academy and enter code: 609003

Effects of Test Anxiety

Test anxiety is like a disease—if left untreated, it will get progressively worse. Anxiety leads to poor performance, and this reinforces the feelings of fear and failure, which in turn lead to poor performances on subsequent tests. It can grow from a mild nervousness to a crippling condition. If allowed to progress, test anxiety can have a big impact on your schooling, and consequently on your future.

Test anxiety can spread to other parts of your life. Anxiety on tests can become anxiety in any stressful situation, and blanking on a test can turn into panicking in a job situation. But fortunately, you don't have to let anxiety rule your testing and determine your grades. There are a number of relatively simple steps you can take to move past anxiety and function normally on a test and in the rest of life.

> **Review Video: How Test Anxiety Impacts Your Grades**
> Visit mometrix.com/academy and enter code: 939819

Physical Steps for Beating Test Anxiety

While test anxiety is a serious problem, the good news is that it can be overcome. It doesn't have to control your ability to think and remember information. While it may take time, you can begin taking steps today to beat anxiety.

Just as your first hint that you may be struggling with anxiety comes from the physical symptoms, the first step to treating it is also physical. Rest is crucial for having a clear, strong mind. If you are tired, it is much easier to give in to anxiety. But if you establish good sleep habits, your body and mind will be ready to perform optimally, without the strain of exhaustion. Additionally, sleeping well helps you to retain information better, so you're more likely to recall the answers when you see the test questions.

Getting good sleep means more than going to bed on time. It's important to allow your brain time to relax. Take study breaks from time to time so it doesn't get overworked, and don't study right before bed. Take time to rest your mind before trying to rest your body, or you may find it difficult to fall asleep.

> **Review Video: The Importance of Sleep for Your Brain**
> Visit mometrix.com/academy and enter code: 319338

Along with sleep, other aspects of physical health are important in preparing for a test. Good nutrition is vital for good brain function. Sugary foods and drinks may give a burst of energy but this burst is followed by a crash, both physically and emotionally. Instead, fuel your body with protein and vitamin-rich foods.

Also, drink plenty of water. Dehydration can lead to headaches and exhaustion, especially if your brain is already under stress from the rigors of the test. Particularly if your test is a long one, drink water during the breaks. And if possible, take an energy-boosting snack to eat between sections.

> **Review Video: How Diet Can Affect your Mood**
> Visit mometrix.com/academy and enter code: 624317

Along with sleep and diet, a third important part of physical health is exercise. Maintaining a steady workout schedule is helpful, but even taking 5-minute study breaks to walk can help get your blood pumping faster and clear your head. Exercise also releases endorphins, which contribute to a positive feeling and can help combat test anxiety.

When you nurture your physical health, you are also contributing to your mental health. If your body is healthy, your mind is much more likely to be healthy as well. So take time to rest, nourish your body with healthy food and water, and get moving as much as possible. Taking these physical steps will make you stronger and more able to take the mental steps necessary to overcome test anxiety.

Review Video: How to Stay Healthy and Prevent Test Anxiety
Visit mometrix.com/academy and enter code: 877894

Mental Steps for Beating Test Anxiety

Working on the mental side of test anxiety can be more challenging, but as with the physical side, there are clear steps you can take to overcome it. As mentioned earlier, test anxiety often stems from lack of preparation, so the obvious solution is to prepare for the test. Effective studying may be the most important weapon you have for beating test anxiety, but you can and should employ several other mental tools to combat fear.

First, boost your confidence by reminding yourself of past success—tests or projects that you aced. If you're putting as much effort into preparing for this test as you did for those, there's no reason you should expect to fail here. Work hard to prepare; then trust your preparation.

Second, surround yourself with encouraging people. It can be helpful to find a study group, but be sure that the people you're around will encourage a positive attitude. If you spend time with others who are anxious or cynical, this will only contribute to your own anxiety. Look for others who are motivated to study hard from a desire to succeed, not from a fear of failure.

Third, reward yourself. A test is physically and mentally tiring, even without anxiety, and it can be helpful to have something to look forward to. Plan an activity following the test, regardless of the outcome, such as going to a movie or getting ice cream.

When you are taking the test, if you find yourself beginning to feel anxious, remind yourself that you know the material. Visualize successfully completing the test. Then take a few deep, relaxing breaths and return to it. Work through the questions carefully but with confidence, knowing that you are capable of succeeding.

Developing a healthy mental approach to test taking will also aid in other areas of life. Test anxiety affects more than just the actual test—it can be damaging to your mental health and even contribute to depression. It's important to beat test anxiety before it becomes a problem for more than testing.

Review Video: Test Anxiety and Depression
Visit mometrix.com/academy and enter code: 904704

Study Strategy

Being prepared for the test is necessary to combat anxiety, but what does being prepared look like? You may study for hours on end and still not feel prepared. What you need is a strategy for test prep. The next few pages outline our recommended steps to help you plan out and conquer the challenge of preparation.

STEP 1: SCOPE OUT THE TEST

Learn everything you can about the format (multiple choice, essay, etc.) and what will be on the test. Gather any study materials, course outlines, or sample exams that may be available. Not only will this help you to prepare, but knowing what to expect can help to alleviate test anxiety.

STEP 2: MAP OUT THE MATERIAL

Look through the textbook or study guide and make note of how many chapters or sections it has. Then divide these over the time you have. For example, if a book has 15 chapters and you have five days to study, you need to cover three chapters each day. Even better, if you have the time, leave an extra day at the end for overall review after you have gone through the material in depth.

If time is limited, you may need to prioritize the material. Look through it and make note of which sections you think you already have a good grasp on, and which need review. While you are studying, skim quickly through the familiar sections and take more time on the challenging parts. Write out your plan so you don't get lost as you go. Having a written plan also helps you feel more in control of the study, so anxiety is less likely to arise from feeling overwhelmed at the amount to cover.

STEP 3: GATHER YOUR TOOLS

Decide what study method works best for you. Do you prefer to highlight in the book as you study and then go back over the highlighted portions? Or do you type out notes of the important information? Or is it helpful to make flashcards that you can carry with you? Assemble the pens, index cards, highlighters, post-it notes, and any other materials you may need so you won't be distracted by getting up to find things while you study.

If you're having a hard time retaining the information or organizing your notes, experiment with different methods. For example, try color-coding by subject with colored pens, highlighters, or post-it notes. If you learn better by hearing, try recording yourself reading your notes so you can listen while in the car, working out, or simply sitting at your desk. Ask a friend to quiz you from your flashcards, or try teaching someone the material to solidify it in your mind.

STEP 4: CREATE YOUR ENVIRONMENT

It's important to avoid distractions while you study. This includes both the obvious distractions like visitors and the subtle distractions like an uncomfortable chair (or a too-comfortable couch that makes you want to fall asleep). Set up the best study environment possible: good lighting and a comfortable work area. If background music helps you focus, you may want to turn it on, but otherwise keep the room quiet. If you are using a computer to take notes, be sure you don't have any other windows open, especially applications like social media, games, or anything else that could distract you. Silence your phone and turn off notifications. Be sure to keep water close by so you stay hydrated while you study (but avoid unhealthy drinks and snacks).

Also, take into account the best time of day to study. Are you freshest first thing in the morning? Try to set aside some time then to work through the material. Is your mind clearer in the afternoon or evening? Schedule your study session then. Another method is to study at the same time of day that you will take the test, so that your brain gets used to working on the material at that time and will be ready to focus at test time.

STEP 5: STUDY!

Once you have done all the study preparation, it's time to settle into the actual studying. Sit down, take a few moments to settle your mind so you can focus, and begin to follow your study plan. Don't give in to distractions or let yourself procrastinate. This is your time to prepare so you'll be ready to fearlessly approach the test. Make the most of the time and stay focused.

Of course, you don't want to burn out. If you study too long you may find that you're not retaining the information very well. Take regular study breaks. For example, taking five minutes out of every hour to walk briskly, breathing deeply and swinging your arms, can help your mind stay fresh.

As you get to the end of each chapter or section, it's a good idea to do a quick review. Remind yourself of what you learned and work on any difficult parts. When you feel that you've mastered the material, move on to the next part. At the end of your study session, briefly skim through your notes again.

But while review is helpful, cramming last minute is NOT. If at all possible, work ahead so that you won't need to fit all your study into the last day. Cramming overloads your brain with more information than it can process and retain, and your tired mind may struggle to recall even previously learned information when it is overwhelmed with last-minute study. Also, the urgent nature of cramming and the stress placed on your brain contribute to anxiety. You'll be more likely to go to the test feeling unprepared and having trouble thinking clearly.

So don't cram, and don't stay up late before the test, even just to review your notes at a leisurely pace. Your brain needs rest more than it needs to go over the information again. In fact, plan to finish your studies by noon or early afternoon the day before the test. Give your brain the rest of the day to relax or focus on other things, and get a good night's sleep. Then you will be fresh for the test and better able to recall what you've studied.

STEP 6: TAKE A PRACTICE TEST

Many courses offer sample tests, either online or in the study materials. This is an excellent resource to check whether you have mastered the material, as well as to prepare for the test format and environment.

Check the test format ahead of time: the number of questions, the type (multiple choice, free response, etc.), and the time limit. Then create a plan for working through them. For example, if you have 30 minutes to take a 60-question test, your limit is 30 seconds per question. Spend less time on the questions you know well so that you can take more time on the difficult ones.

If you have time to take several practice tests, take the first one open book, with no time limit. Work through the questions at your own pace and make sure you fully understand them. Gradually work up to taking a test under test conditions: sit at a desk with all study materials put away and set a timer. Pace yourself to make sure you finish the test with time to spare and go back to check your answers if you have time.

After each test, check your answers. On the questions you missed, be sure you understand why you missed them. Did you misread the question (tests can use tricky wording)? Did you forget the information? Or was it something you hadn't learned? Go back and study any shaky areas that the practice tests reveal.

Taking these tests not only helps with your grade, but also aids in combating test anxiety. If you're already used to the test conditions, you're less likely to worry about it, and working through tests until you're scoring well gives you a confidence boost. Go through the practice tests until you feel comfortable, and then you can go into the test knowing that you're ready for it.

Test Tips

On test day, you should be confident, knowing that you've prepared well and are ready to answer the questions. But aside from preparation, there are several test day strategies you can employ to maximize your performance.

First, as stated before, get a good night's sleep the night before the test (and for several nights before that, if possible). Go into the test with a fresh, alert mind rather than staying up late to study.

Try not to change too much about your normal routine on the day of the test. It's important to eat a nutritious breakfast, but if you normally don't eat breakfast at all, consider eating just a protein bar. If you're a coffee drinker, go ahead and have your normal coffee. Just make sure you time it so that the caffeine doesn't wear off right in the middle of your test. Avoid sugary beverages, and drink enough water to stay hydrated but not so much that you need a restroom break 10 minutes into the test. If your test isn't first thing in the morning, consider going for a walk or doing a light workout before the test to get your blood flowing.

Allow yourself enough time to get ready, and leave for the test with plenty of time to spare so you won't have the anxiety of scrambling to arrive in time. Another reason to be early is to select a good seat. It's helpful to sit away from doors and windows, which can be distracting. Find a good seat, get out your supplies, and settle your mind before the test begins.

When the test begins, start by going over the instructions carefully, even if you already know what to expect. Make sure you avoid any careless mistakes by following the directions.

Then begin working through the questions, pacing yourself as you've practiced. If you're not sure on an answer, don't spend too much time on it, and don't let it shake your confidence. Either skip it and come back later, or eliminate as many wrong answers as possible and guess among the remaining ones. Don't dwell on these questions as you continue—put them out of your mind and focus on what lies ahead.

Be sure to read all of the answer choices, even if you're sure the first one is the right answer. Sometimes you'll find a better one if you keep reading. But don't second-guess yourself if you do immediately know the answer. Your gut instinct is usually right. Don't let test anxiety rob you of the information you know.

If you have time at the end of the test (and if the test format allows), go back and review your answers. Be cautious about changing any, since your first instinct tends to be correct, but make sure you didn't misread any of the questions or accidentally mark the wrong answer choice. Look over any you skipped and make an educated guess.

At the end, leave the test feeling confident. You've done your best, so don't waste time worrying about your performance or wishing you could change anything. Instead, celebrate the successful completion of this test. And finally, use this test to learn how to deal with anxiety even better next time.

> **Review Video: 5 Tips to Beat Test Anxiety**
> Visit mometrix.com/academy and enter code: 570656

Important Qualification

Not all anxiety is created equal. If your test anxiety is causing major issues in your life beyond the classroom or testing center, or if you are experiencing troubling physical symptoms related to your anxiety, it may be a sign of a serious physiological or psychological condition. If this sounds like your situation, we strongly encourage you to seek professional help.

Thank You

We at Mometrix would like to extend our heartfelt thanks to you, our friend and patron, for allowing us to play a part in your journey. It is a privilege to serve people from all walks of life who are unified in their commitment to building the best future they can for themselves.

The preparation you devote to these important testing milestones may be the most valuable educational opportunity you have for making a real difference in your life. We encourage you to put your heart into it—that feeling of succeeding, overcoming, and yes, conquering will be well worth the hours you've invested.

We want to hear your story, your struggles and your successes, and if you see any opportunities for us to improve our materials so we can help others even more effectively in the future, please share that with us as well. **The team at Mometrix would be absolutely thrilled to hear from you!** So please, send us an email (support@mometrix.com) and let's stay in touch.

> **If you'd like some additional help, check out these other resources we offer for your exam:**
> **http://MometrixFlashcards.com/ARDMS**

Additional Bonus Material

Due to our efforts to try to keep this book to a manageable length, we've created a link that will give you access to all of your additional bonus material.

> **Please visit**
> **https://www.mometrix.com/bonus948/ardmsultra**
> **phy to access the information.**